Accession no.
01049471

Fundamentals of Anaesthesia and Acute Medicine

616.0472 RAW 2500
2

JET LIBRARY

Management of Acute and Chronic Pain

Fundamentals of Anaesthesia and Acute Medicine

Management of Acute and Chronic Pain

Edited by
Narinder Rawal
Senior Consultant, Department of Anaesthesiology and Intensive Care, Örebro, Sweden
Visiting Professor, Department of Anesthesiology, University of Texas Medical School, Houston, USA

Series editors
Ronald M Jones
Professor of Anaesthetics, St Mary's Hospital Medical School, London, UK

Alan R Aitkenhead
Professor of Anaesthesia, University of Nottingham, UK

and

Pierre Foëx
Nuffield Professor of Anaesthetics, University of Oxford, UK

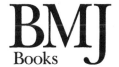

© BMJ Books 1998
BMJ Books is an imprint of the BMJ Publishing Group

All rights reserved. No part of this publication may be reproduced, stored in a retrieval system, or transmitted, in any form or by any means, electronic, mechanical, photocopying recording and/or otherwise, without the prior written permission of the publishers.

First published in 1998
by BMJ Books, BMA House, Tavistock Square,
London WC1H 9JR

British Library Cataloguing in Publication Data

A catalogue record for this book is available from the British Library

ISBN 0-7279-1193-7

Typeset by Apek Typesetters Ltd, Nailsea, Bristol
Printed and bound in Great Britain by Latimer Trend Ltd, Plymouth

Contents

Contributors

Robert Atcheson, MB BS, MD, FRCA
Senior Lecturer and Honorary Consultant in Pain Management and Anaesthesia, University of Leicester and Leicester Royal Infirmary, UK

Anders Ekblom, MD, PhD, DDS
Department of Anesthesiology and Intensive Care, Karolinska Hospital/Institute, Stockholm, Sweden; Concept Division, Astra Pain Control AB, Södertälje, Sweden

Isabelle Murat, MD, PhD
Professor of Anaesthesiology and Intensive Care, Service d'Anesthésie-Réanimation, Hôpital Armand Trousseau, Paris, France

Richard B Patt, MD
Associate Professor of Anesthesiology and Neuro-oncology, Director of Anesthesia Pain Programs and Fellowship, and Deputy Chief of Pain and Symptom Management Section, University of Texas MD Anderson Cancer Center, Houston, Texas, USA

Prithvi Raj, MD, FACPM
Professor and Co-director, Pain Services, Texas Tech University Health Sciences Center, Lubbock, Texas, USA

Richard L Rauck, MD
Director, Pain Control Center and Associate Professor of Anesthesia, Wake Forest University Medical Center, Winston Salem, North Carolina, USA

Narinder Rawal, MD, PhD
Senior Consultant, Department of Anesthesiology and Intensive Care, Örebro Medical Center Hospital, Örebro, Sweden; Visiting Professor, Department of Anesthesiology, University of Texas Medical School, Houston, Texas, USA

Suresh Reddy, MD, FFARCS
Junior Faculty Associate, Anesthesiology Pain Management, University of Texas MD Anderson Cancer Center, Houston, Texas, USA

David J Rowbotham, MB, ChB, MD, MRCP, FRCA
Professor and Honorary Consultant in Pain Management and Anaesthesia, University of Leicester and Leicester Royal Infirmary, UK

Malin Rydh-Rinder, MD
Department of Neuroscience, Karolinska Institute, Stockholm, Sweden; Preclinical Research and Development, Astra Pain Control AB, Södertälje, Sweden

André van Zundert, MD, PhD
Department of Anesthesiology, Intensive Care and Pain Therapy, Catharina Hospital, Eindhoven, The Netherlands

Foreword

The Fundamentals of Anaesthesia and Acute Medicine Series

The pace of change within the biological sciences continues to increase and nowhere is this more apparent than in the specialties of anaesthesia, acute medicine, and intensive care. Although many practitioners continue to rely on comprehensive but bulky texts for reference, the accelerating rate of biomedical advances makes this source of information increasingly likely to be dated, even if the latest edition is used. The series *Fundamentals of Anaesthesia and Acute Medicine* aims to bring to the reader up to date and authoritative reviews of the principal clinical topics which make up the specialties. Each volume will cover the fundamentals of the topic in a comprehensive manner but will also emphasise recent developments of controversial issues.

International differences in the practice of anaesthesia and intensive care are now much less than in the past, and the editors of each volume have commissioned chapters from acknowledged authorities throughout the world to assemble contributions of the highest possible calibre. Three volumes will appear annually and, as the pace and extent of clinically significant advances varies among the individual topics, new editions will be commissioned to ensure that practitioners will be in a position to keep abreast of the important developments within the specialties.

Not only does the pace of advance in biomedical science serve to justify the appearance of an international series of this nature but the current awareness of the need for more formal continuing education also underlines the timeliness of its appearance. The editors would welcome feedback from readers about the series, which is aimed at both established practitioners and trainees preparing for degrees and diplomas in anaesthesia and intensive care.

RONALD M JONES
ALAN R AITKENHEAD
PIERRE FOËX

Preface

Relieving pain has always been one of the major aims of the medical profession but it has also been one of the most elusive. Although the means have been available for several decades, adequate treatment of pain has generally been neglected. Untreated pain causes physical and mental changes by destroying sleep, impairing tissue function, and sometimes causing depression. However, in recent years interest in pain management has increased dramatically. This is based on enormous advances in the development of basic research in the study of pain and its application in clinical practice. In some countries a new subspecialty of pain medicine has been created. The discovery of opioid receptors paved the way for spinal opioid analgesia which has been revolutionary in the management of cancer, obstetric, and postoperative pain. The concept of patient controlled analgesia has also achieved widespread acceptance. Increasingly acute pain teams are being established to facilitate the use of these special techniques.

The aim of this book is to provide doctors in training, and medical practitioners, with recent advances in pain management. Throughout the text the approach is clinical with contributions from a group of internationally recognised specialists who emphasise most of the major issues in pain management. These experts explore a variety of important issues including anatomy, physiology, and pharmacology of pain as well as the management of acute (postoperative, obstetric, paediatric), chronic, and cancer pain. Newer drugs, interventional modalities, and drug delivery techniques such as epidural, spinal, patient controlled analgesia are highlighted. It is hoped that the material presented in the following chapters will be useful to the clinician who manages pain patients.

The success of any multiauthored book is in large part dependent on the expertise of the contributors and the extent of their commitment. The contributors to this book are acknowledged authorities in their respective fields; without their support this book would not exist. They have my sincere thanks. I am grateful for the help and flexibility provided by the staff of BMJ Books, especially Mary Banks, during the entire project.

Narinder Rawal

1: Pain mechanisms: anatomy and physiology

ANDERS EKBLOM and MALIN RYDH-RINDER

Introductory comments

This chapter focuses on the physiological and pathophysiological mechanisms of pain, with only limited data on traditional anatomy. For a more thorough description of peripheral and central nervous structures of importance for pain perception, the reader is referred to textbooks on relevant anatomy and especially neuroanatomy. Primarily physiological and nociceptive pain will be considered, with reference to other chapters for a discussion of neurogenic or neuropathic pain, including the importance of the sympathetic nervous system.

Several diseases include pain as an important feature alerting the patient to take action. Pain as a symptom is often used by the physician in establishing the diagnosis. Pain is, however, part of normal physiology, providing the individual with a warning system of vital importance for survival. This is illustrated by the risk of tissue injury and disease resulting in increased morbidity and mortality in patients with congenital pain insensitivity or analgesia. Patients with various neuropathies are a group at risk due to decreased sensory sensitivity.

Pain can roughly be divided into at least two types, physiological and clinical. The former is due to the activation of nociceptive afferent nerve fibres, a group responding to potentially tissue-damaging or noxious stimuli. Activity in the nociceptive afferents is transmitted to the central nervous system (CNS) and may result in reflex responses and the sensation of pain. Physiological pain is normally of short duration and represents a warning system for potentially harmful stimuli.

In contrast, clinical pain or pain due to pathology or injury, is related to activation of the nociceptive afferents as part of a disease or trauma. It is then termed nociceptive pain. If pain is the result from injury or lesions of the peripheral and/or the central nervous system, it may be called neurogenic or neuropathic pain. The analysis of pain with respect to basic mechanisms has proved to be of value in establishing a firm diagnosis and when deciding upon appropriate treatment.

1

Clinical knowledge thus suggests that different physiological and pathophysiological mechanisms explain pain in different clinical conditions. Further, it is improbable that one single universal treatment is to be found for all kinds of pain. Instead it seems reasonable to seek these different mechanisms. Peripheral mechanisms, central mechanisms, and endogenous pain-controlling mechanisms will be considered.

Peripheral mechanisms

The primary sensory neuron

The primary sensory neuron is the first cell to transmit information from the periphery to the spinal cord. Its cell body is located in the dorsal root ganglion (DRG) and its axon consists of a peripheral and a central branch (Fig. 1.1). This nerve cell is a pseudounipolar neuron and the cell body is not directly involved in the synaptic transmission of the signal. This anatomical feature permits the neuron to exert effects in the periphery as well as in the central nervous system.

Sensory nerve fibres are classified as A- and C-fibres depending on diameter and whether they are sheathed with myelin. A-fibres are myelinated and have the larger diameters. The sensory population can further be divided into Aβ- and Aδ-fibres according to size (Table 1.1).

A-fibres

Aδ-fibres are the thinnest myelinated fibres, and are involved in nociception and pain (and cold) sensations. As the conduction speed is

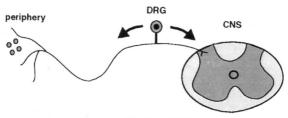

Fig 1.1 Primary sensory afferent with its cell body located in the dorsal root ganglion (DRG)

Table 1.1 Classification of afferent fibres

Sensory fibre type	Fibre diameter (μm)	Conduction velocity (m/s)
Aβ	6–12	35–75
Aδ	1–5	5–30
C	0·2–1·5	0·1–2

higher than in C-fibres, these fibres are thought to mediate the first pain response following, for example, skin stimulation of an extremity. The early pain response following a defined stimulation of the skin is perceived as distinct and well localised.

Activation of $A\beta$-fibres evokes non-painful sensations (touch, pressure, vibration) from both muscles and skin under normal conditions. However, $A\beta$ stimulation may provoke pain in inflammatory pain states and in some pathological neurogenic pain states.

C-fibres

C-fibres are unmyelinated and thin, resulting in a slower conduction velocity than A-fibres. The majority of C-fibres may be involved in pain and nociception, although activity in other fibres results in non-painful sensations (warmth, itch). C-fibre-mediated pain following cutaneous stimulation has a more diffuse and dull quality.

Glial cells

Nerve cells and glial cells exist in close relation to each other and interact in many respects. Schwann cells represent glial cells present both in the DRG and in the periphery, while satellite cells are only found in the DRG. One important function of Schwann cells is the production of myelin folded around the nerve fibres, which gives a faster, saltatoric propagation of action potentials along the nerve. Unmyelinated fibres are covered only by protecting Schwann cells. The glia gives the nerve mechanical support, guides axonal growth, and is also important for transmitter metabolism, nutrition, and blood–brain barrier function. After tissue damage the glial cells also exhibit phagocytotic properties.

Nociceptors and nociceptive afferents

In the various tissues of the body different receptors and innervating fibres provide the peripheral basis for somatosensory functions. The receptors have different sensitivities towards different kinds of stimuli. Those activated by stimuli threatening tissue integrity are called nociceptors. The nociceptors are considered to be the distal ends of the free naked nerve endings of the $A\delta$- and C-fibre nociceptive afferents.

There are more C-fibres then $A\delta$-fibres. Due to their small diameter, nociceptors cannot be directly recorded from, only indirectly through the parent nerve fibres. Nociceptors and nociceptive afferents are classified by fibre type ($A\delta$-, myelinated- and C-, unmyelinated fibre) and according to the stimuli that activate them (mechanical, thermal, and chemical). Thus, for example, there are A-MH units ($A\delta$-, mechano-heat-sensitive fibres) or C-polymodal units (C-, mechano-heat-chemically sensitive fibres). Since different classes of nociceptive afferents may be found, based on stimulus-response characteristics, this should correspond to membrane receptor specialisations of the naked nerve endings. No specific receptor structures are, however, visible with traditional morphological techniques.

Nociceptive fibres are usually bi- or polymodal with respect to their adequate stimuli. An additional, newly described group of fibres is the "silent" or "sleeping" fibres. These are not (easily) recruited by mechanical or thermal stimuli in normal tissues but they become excitable following local inflammation. They may be of importance following inflammation and trauma, participating in the development of hyperalgesia and neurogenic inflammation.

Inflammation, pain-provoking substances, and peripheral sensitisation

Various substances produced during inflammation can directly activate the nociceptive afferents, sensitise them, and/or result in release of proinflammatory substances from them.

Direct activation of nociceptive afferents

Several substances activate nociceptive afferents in various tissues, following application locally or injected into blood vessels very near the receptive fields. Examples of endogenously produced or released substances are acetylcholine, adenosine, bradykinin, histamine, serotonin, and protons and K^+ ions. Recent research has clearly demonstrated a receptor selectivity with respect to activation of algogenic substances on nociceptors and afferents.

An ingredient of Spanish pepper, capsaicin, produces intense burning pain following cutaneous application in humans, an action provoked through the activation of nociceptive C-fibres. Capsaicin has gained interest due to this specific effect on C-fibres, and recent data suggest the action to be receptor specific. In fact, a specific antagonist, capsazepine, has been developed. The natural ligand for the capsaicin receptor is suggested by some to be H^+ ions. Following cutaneous injection with capsaicin, humans experience intense burning pain but also thermal hyperalgesia (increased pain intensity perceived following a normally painful heat stimulus) at the injection site, later followed by hypoalgesia to pain. A zone of allodynia to touch (normal touch stimuli perceived as painful) develops around the capsaicin-injected area as does a zone of cutaneous flare. The hyperalgesia is due to peripheral sensitisation of the nociceptive afferents, whereas the allodynia is due to central changes in the spinal cord.

Peripheral sensitisation of nociceptive afferents

During inflammation for example, prostaglandins and leukotrienes are produced through the action of cyclooxygenase (COX) and lipoxygenase, respectively. Some of these substances can increase the sensitivity of the nociceptors and nociceptive afferents towards other pain-producing substances or stimuli (thermal, mechanical, and chemical stimulation for $A\delta$- and C-fibres, the former of special importance in glabrous skin). Prostaglandins (PGE_1 and PGE_2) can significantly increase the sensitivity of nociceptive afferents to bradykinin. Similar data have been presented for leukotrienes (LTB_4). Recently, two isoforms of COX have been described as being of importance for prostaglandin synthesis. COX-1 is constitutively expressed in several tissues but COX-2 is induced only during inflammation. Animal data have been presented where COX-2 inhibitors reduce nociception and inflammation while initial clinical data document a reduction of postoperative pain. The possibility of developing non-steroidal anti-inflammatory drugs (NSAIDs) without the side-effects of today's drugs is therefore very interesting.

It seems as if there is a significant synergy between various combinations of substances producing peripheral sensitisation, for example prostaglandins and bradykinin. A result of afferents being sensitised is primary hyperalgesia. An important mechanism for primary afferent hyperalgesia is that the algogenic substances increase second-messenger systems such as intracellular cAMP through stimulatory G-proteins (G_s). In injured or inflamed skin a decreased pain threshold can be found as well as increased pain intensity following a normally painful stimulus. Spontaneous pain may also be reported (Table 1.2).

Peptidergic release from nociceptive afferents

Approximately 80% of the peptides produced in the cell bodies of the afferents is transposed to the periphery. This efferent pool of peptides may be released in response to nerve activation, directly or through axon reflexes in branching fibres. Following release, the peptides take part in the inflammatory process (Fig. 1.2). The term neurogenic inflammation indicates that the peptides may participate in reactions resulting in the signs of inflammation such as redness, heat, swelling, and pain. Once the peptides are released they may stimulate various inflammatory cells to release proinflammatory substances, creating a vicious feed-forward circle. Several animal studies have shown that depletion of neuropeptides in afferent fibres significantly reduces the inflammatory reactions. A trophic role for some of the peptides has also been suggested.

Table 1.2 Characteristics of sensitisation and primary hyperalgesia

Sensitisation (electrophysiological findings)	Primary hyperalgesia (psychophysical data)
Decreased threshold for activation	Decreased pain threshold
Increased nerve impulse frequency at stimulation	Increased pain intensity at stimulation
Spontaneous nerve impulse activity	Spontaneous pain

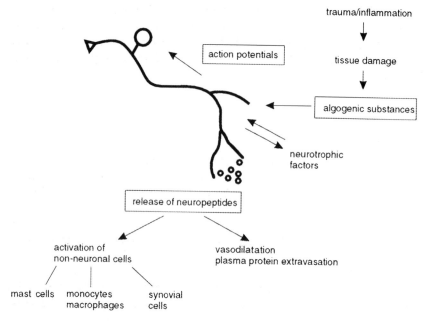

Fig 1.2   Afferent and efferent aspects of a peptidergic nociceptive afferent fibre

Neurotrophins and especially nerve growth factor (NGF) are produced by peripheral cells such as fibroblasts and Schwann cells. NGF is of vital importance for the survival of afferents as well as for maintaining their phenotype. Cytokines, such as some of the interleukins, released from inflammatory cells may stimulate expression of NGF which would explain their hyperalgesic effects. Interestingly, NGF may increase the production of neuropeptides and influence expression of sodium channels in the nociceptive afferents, and thereby influence inflammatory hypersensitivity. The receptor through which NGF may interact on nociceptive afferents is a tyrosine kinase A receptor called trkA.

Classification of DRG neurons

DRG neurons can roughly be discriminated according to cell size and morphology. The description of large, light cells and small, dark neurons is commonly used. However, a considerable number of intermediate-sized neurons also exist in the DRG. The classical view suggests C-fibre afferents are connected to small dark neurons, whereas neurons with axons in the $A\delta$ range predominantly have cell bodies of intermediate size. The large, light cells are considered to be associated with fast-conducting fibres of $A\alpha$ and $A\beta$ types.

How the sensory information is transmitted from these cells to the spinal cord neurons has been a scientific issue for many years. The chemical profile of DRG neurons has been extensively studied. DRG neurons do not express acetylcholine or amines which are important transmitters in the autonomic nervous system. The DRG produces a number of peptides as well as amino acids which can thus be considered as putative neurotransmitters.

Central mechanisms

Spinal cord

The cord is divided into cervical, thoracic, lumbar and sacral parts. Two enlargements, one in the cervical and the other in the lumbar part, accommodate the innervation of the limbs. The ventral and dorsal roots join together just distally to the DRG to form a mixed spinal nerve consisting of afferent as well as efferent nerve fibres (Fig. 1.3). The spinal cord can be segmentally divided corresponding to each pair of spinal nerves that is formed and emerges from each intervertebral foramen. There are eight cervical, 12 thoracic, five lumbar, and five sacral spinal nerves.

The spinal cord itself is composed of white and grey matter. The white matter consists mainly of nerve bundles and supporting glial elements, while the central grey matter consists mainly of cell bodies.

The proportion of white matter to grey increases in the upper parts because of the addition of axons along the way up to the brain stem. The proportion of grey matter is highest in the lower region; as the limbs and trunk require a larger number of motor- and interneurons many descending axons have terminated higher up. The white matter is divided into three bilateral and paired columns or funiculi. The dorsal column forms one of the major ascending systems for sensory information. The lateral columns

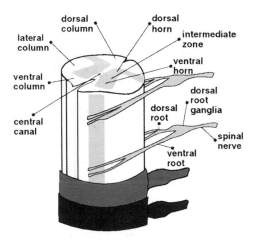

Fig 1.3 Key anatomical features of the spinal cord and peripheral nerves

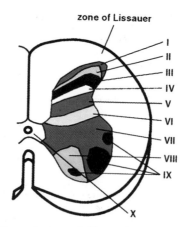

Fig 1.4 Section of the spinal cord illustrating the localisation of the Rexed laminae

contain both ascending sensory pathways and descending control systems from the brain, while the ventral column is formed by axons derived from the motor neurons in the ventral horn. The grey matter can be divided into a ventral and a dorsal horn with an intermediate zone in between.

A laminar organisation of the spinal grey matter in the cat was suggested in 1952 by Bror Rexed (Fig. 1.4). His classification was based on 10 laminae and this was later shown to correspond well to cell clusters or spinal cord nuclei with different functions. This classification also seems useful for other species including humans (Table 1.3).

Afferent fibres enter the spinal cord via the dorsal root. Large diameter fibres mediating tactile and proprioceptive information reach the grey matter via the medial aspect of the dorsal horn and terminate in the nucleus proprius (laminae III–IV). Fibres of small diameter conveying pain and temperature enter via the zone of Lissauer, located dorsolaterally to lamina I in the dorsal horn. After passing this entry zone these fibres spread to nearby levels before they enter and terminate in the outer regions such as laminae I, II, and III. Myelinated small diameter fibres (Aδ) form synapses in the outermost layer, lamina I, as well as in the nucleus proprius.

Neurotransmitters and modulators

Three classes of neurotransmitter, namely peptides, amino acids, and the nitric oxide (NO) gas molecule, have been found in primary sensory neurons. Considering the efferent function of sensory nerves they may also be looked upon as a potential source of peripheral mediators in inflammatory processes. Some of them are important for excitatory mechanisms whereas others participate in the equally important endogenous inhibitory processes.

Table 1.3   Laminar arrangement of the spinal cord grey matter

Laminae	Region	Nuclei	Function
I	Dorsal horn	Marginal zone	Outer area of dorsal horn Processes pain and temperature sense
II	Dorsal horn	Substantia gelatinosa	Receives input from C-fibre afferents, hence important station for pain and sensory transmission
III–VI	Dorsal horn	Nucleus proprius	Deeper laminae processing sensory and nociceptive information with descending pathways
VII	Intermediate zone	Clarke's nucleus (T1–L2) Intermediolateral/ medial nuclei	Proprioceptive transmission Nuclei involved in the autonomic nervous system
VIII	Ventral horn		Cutaneous and proprioceptive input
IX	Ventral horn	Motor nuclei	Large α-motor neurons innervating skeletal muscle
X	Around the central canal		Some cells responding to noxious stimuli

Substance P (SP)

SP is probably the best studied peptide today and is widely distributed in the peripheral and central nervous system. There is now a large body of evidence that SP is important in nociception. SP is mainly produced in small DRG neurons which are connected to C-fibres. In the spinal dorsal horn a dense network of SP-positive nerve fibres is concentrated in laminae I and II, where partial processing of nociception takes place. When injected intrathecally in rats, SP evokes scratching, biting, and licking thought to be correlated to pain sensations. SP acts as an excitatory peptide on a subpopulation of dorsal horn neurons when applied ionthophoretically. It is also found in spinal interneurons and descending pathways and might therefore be important in various control systems. SP belongs to the tachykinin family together with neurokinin A (NKA) and neurokinin B (NKB). They act on specific NK-receptors which can be further divided into NK1-, NK2- and NK3-receptors, with SP, NKA, and NKB as the respective preferred ligands. NKA seems to resemble SP. Both these tachykinins are produced by DRG neurons, and are released upon noxious stimulation and may activate the same type of receptor (NK1-receptors), although they are not equipotent. NK1-receptor antagonists exert presumed analgesic effects in several animals. NKB is, in contrast to SP and NKA, not found in DRG cells.

Calictonin gene-related peptide (CGRP)

CGRP is also an excitatory peptide, discovered some 50 years later (1982) than SP. In virtually all SP neurons coexistence with CGRP can be demonstrated. This peptide also coexists with a number of other peptides in DRG neurons, such as galanin (GAL), vasoactive intestinal peptide (VIP), somatostatin (SOM), cholecystokinin (CCK), and dynorphin (DYN).

CGRP exerts synergistic effects with SP when applied simultaneously to the spinal cord. It prolongs the nociceptive-related behaviour induced by SP. In peripheral tissues CGRP exhibits a very potent vasodilatory capacity which may also contribute to the flare reaction seen in peripheral inflammation.

Somatostatin (SOM)

SOM was discovered in 1973 and was later localised in both the peripheral and central nervous systems. In the DRG, a subpopulation of sensory neurons expresses SOM and a small number of these also express SP. Virtually all SOM neurons also seem to contain CGRP. In the spinal cord, SOM-containing terminals are found in the dorsal horn, predominantly in lamina II. However, not more than 20% of spinal SOM are of sensory origin. The response to intrathecally injected SOM is very similar to that of SP, mimicking a peripheral noxious stimulus. SOM is also released from primary afferents after mechanical and heat stimulation of the skin. However, no changes in experimental nociception and pain behaviour were observed after selective chemical depletion of SOM in animal studies. In fact SOM has been looked upon as a potential antinociceptive substance due to its inhibitory function in the spinal cord. SOM has been tried epidurally, in mainly postoperative clinical conditions, but no significant effect has been documented and in fact animal studies have indicated a clear risk of neurotoxicity (motor dysfunction, paralysis).

Vasoactive intestinal peptide (VIP)

Another peptide with potent vasodilatory action is VIP, which is also extensively distributed in the peripheral and central nervous systems. VIP is found in DRG neurons in some cases coexisting with SP and, spinally, mainly in lamina I. Noxious levels of electrical stimulation induce release of VIP which can increase excitability and depolarise dorsal horn cells. However, VIP is not considered to be normally a sensory transmitter of great importance although in the autonomic nervous system it is an important co-transmitter with acetylcholine. After peripheral nerve lesions, however, VIP is upregulated in sensory neurons and may have an extended role in neurotransmission during neuropathic pain.

Galanin (GAL)

GAL is a peptide with inhibitory properties. In the normal state a few DRG neurons, mainly small, express the peptide. GAL has been suggested to be of importance during neuronal injuries when it is dramatically upregulated in DRG neurons in many species. Experimental sciatic nerve section is one experimental model for studies of neuropathic pain states in animals. It induces licking and biting of the engaged limb. In the rat some 50% of the animals exhibit the self-mutilation termed autotomy following nerve injury. Intrathecal treatment with a GAL receptor antagonist after this type of nerve lesion induced more severe autotomy in rats. These results point to an endogenous controlling role for GAL in neuropathic pain states perhaps by inhibiting pathological excitation.

Cholecystokinin (CCK)

CCK can be found in various parts of the CNS including spinal neurons. Animal research has shown that the spinal application of CCK antagonises the analgesic action of morphine, and the administration of a CCK_B antagonist may enhance morphine analgesia. Interestingly, a decreased concentration of CCK during inflammation may underlie the effectiveness of opioids in these situations. In experimental models of neuropathic pain CCK is upregulated, which could explain the relative decrease in analgesic efficacy of opioids, bearing a resemblance to the opioid resistance in neuropathic pain discussed in patients.

It is interesting to note that the CCK system could represent a mechanism for the modulation of efficacy of the endogenous opioid system, at least with respect to μ-receptor-mediated analgesia.

Purines

Adenosine triphosphate (ATP) was described to be released from primary afferents in the periphery. When cell damage occurs, ATP may leak out in the tissue and lead to afferent nerve activation. It was later shown to be released within the dorsal horn. The exact location and origin still remain to be confirmed. ATP released from nerves is known to act at a P2X subtype of P2 purinoceptors. The functional receptor is a heteromeric assembly of different subunits. It has recently been shown that C-fibre afferents express a specific receptor subunit called P2X3. This may lead to the discovery of yet another site-specific target for pharmacological intervention against pain. A subset of dorsal horn neurons is depolarised by ATP. This finding provides further evidence for ATP being one important candidate in fast sensory transmission in the spinal dorsal horn but also a possible peripheral mediator in pain signalling.

Adenosine is generated during hypoxia and activates C-fibres and induces nociceptive behaviour in animals. Local cutaneous or intra-arterial application in humans provokes the sensation of pain. In animal studies, the excitatory action on peripheral afferents seems to be mediated through activation of A_2-receptors.

Interestingly, in animal studies, the activation of spinal A_1-receptors correlates with inhibitory effects on spinal neurons through hyper-polarisation and antinociceptive effects following intrathecal administration. Thus the administration route and type of adenosine receptor activated result in opposite effects, as seen with other substances such as serotonin (5-HT). More recent data in humans suggest an analgesic effect of adenosine given intravenously or intrathecally.

Excitatory amino acids

A number of studies have provided evidence that glutamate (GLU) is a major excitatory sensory transmitter. GLU has been shown by immunohistochemistry to be present in C-fibre afferents and DRGs, often co-localised with SP. Several studies have proved that it is released in the spinal cord following peripheral noxious stimulation or following nerve activation. Excitatory amino acids (EAA) act on a number of receptors. GLU depolarises spinal cord neurons via voltage-gated ion-channel coupled receptors, but may also act at metabotropic- or G-protein-coupled receptors. In a pain perspective most interest so far has been in the ion-channel coupled receptors, as they seem to be involved in sensory transmission. They mediate fast excitatory postsynaptic potentials and can be divided roughly into N-methyl-D-aspartate- (NMDA) and non-NMDA-receptors. Non-NMDA-receptors are further classified into quisqualate-(AMPA) and kainate-receptors according to their most selective ligand. The NMDA-receptor is of great interest for both acute and chronic pain states. Studies have shown a distinct concentration of NMDA-receptor binding sites in the superficial layers of the dorsal horn, areas known to be involved in pain transmission. There is substantial evidence that GLU can depolarise dorsal horn neurons and potentiate responses from these upon noxious stimuli. Blocking NMDA-receptors prevents the characteristic increase in response, the "wind-up" phenomenon, seen in dorsal horn neurons following repeated constant-intensity stimulation of C-fibres. Pain-related behaviour in animals can be evoked by intrathecal administration of EAAs which can be counteracted by the use of NMDA-receptor-antagonists.

In a number of studies using animal behavioural models, EAA antagonists have exhibited antinociceptive properties. There is some experience from using non-competitive NMDA antagonists such as ketamine in humans. In experimentally induced pain in human volunteers, the NMDA antagonists ketamine or dextrorphan reduced pain due to lowered central summation of nociceptive afferent activity and reduced central sensitisation. In patients both acute nociceptive pain and chronic neuropathic pain (e.g. post herpetic neuralgia) are decreased following systemically administered ketamine. A direct spinal pain-reducing effect has been reported in a study documenting the effect of intrathecally given 3-(2-carboxypiperazin-4-yl) propyl-phosphonic acid (CPP) in a patient with chronic neuropathic pain. Interestingly, heat pain perception was unchanged but some components of the neuropathic pain were attenuated.

NMDA-receptor antagonists may have a role in antinociception and analgesia but this remains to be fully clinically established.

Nitric oxide (NO)

NO was first believed to be an endothelial factor called endothelial-derived-relaxing factor (EDRF), but was later shown to be the small NO molecule, synthesised by an enzyme, nitric oxide synthase (NOS), from the amino acid L-arginine which is expressed in a variety of cell types and not only in the endothelium. NOS has been demonstrated in both peripheral and central neurons, which led to the suggestion that NO may be of importance in neuronal signalling. Bradykinin activates afferent C-fibres and is an important mediator in peripheral inflammation. Bradykinin induces NO production and there is some evidence NO is released from neurons after receptor activation. NMDA-receptor activation leads to stimulation of guanylate cyclase, which seems to be mediated via generation of NO. The NMDA-receptor may be important in pain and nociception involving NO. Taken together, these facts highlight NO as a possible mediator in painful processes. A few primary sensory neurons express NOS in normal situations, but after nerve injury NOS is dramatically increased in DRG neurons, which might indicate a specific role for NO in neuropathic pain or nerve regeneration. Intravenous, local or intrathecal administration of a NO inhibitor results in antinociceptive effects in a classic model of inflammatory pain, the formalin test. The results suggest that NO is active both at the peripheral site of activation and at the spinal level. In contrast, local application of the NO precursor L-arginine reduced pain-related behaviour in the formalin test. For this reason the role of NO in, especially, peripheral nociceptive mechanisms is debatable.

Nociceptive neurons in the spinal cord

The dorsal horn of the spinal cord represents the first site for synaptic transmission of afferent activity to the second-order neurons. In general, these neurons can be divided into two types, the nociceptive specific (NS) and the wide-dynamic-range (WDR) neuron (Fig. 1.5). The NS neuron is only activated by high-threshold nociceptive afferents and has a small receptive field. NS neurons are mainly confined to the outermost part of the

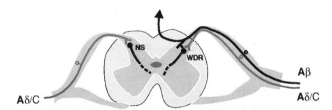

Fig 1.5   NS and WDR neurons are found in the dorsal horn of the spinal cord

dorsal horn. WDR neurons are multireceptive, since they respond to activation of afferent fibres conveying mechanical, thermal and noxious information. In lamina V a majority of nociceptive afferents contact this type of second-order neuron. The WDR neurons have a large receptive field and animal studies suggest that they are important for sensory discriminative input due to their response characteristics. This is, however, not a static situation, since the NS neuron may reversibly change into a WDR neuron during certain conditions. Repetitive C-fibre stimulation induces changes in the receptive field of the dorsal horn neuron within a minute, which suggests that some synapses may be normally silent or functionally inefficient but are recruited during special circumstances. Nociceptive fibres also terminate in a highly ordered way. Different fibre types end up in different laminae and different body areas are represented topographically. Nociceptive transmission in the spinal cord includes interneurons modulating pain responses and ventral horn motoneurons evoking spinal reflexes, which are important protective mechanisms.

Neuronal responses in the dorsal horn to sensory activation consist of both a fast and a slow component. The excitatory amino acids, especially glutamate but also purines such as ATP, have been proposed as fast transmitters and the peptides, in general, as more slow and modulatory components. Taken together the spinal cord neurons, like the peripheral neurons, exhibit a dynamic plasticity which gives rise to a broad range of responses and a large variation of pain processing in the sensory nervous system. This plasticity is being increasingly recognised and indicates therapeutic challenges and possibilities.

A mechanism thought to be dependent on spinal mechanisms is referred pain. It is clinically well known that pain from deep somatic and visceral structures may be localised to distant structures. One often cited example is patients with angina pectoris or myocardial infarction localising their pain and discomfort to the anterior chest, parts of the left arm, or even the lower jaw. The area for referral may become tender and hyperalgesia may develop over time. Several typical clinical conditions exist, suggesting that the phenomenon of referred pain is due to some common physiological mechanism. One early proposal was based on the finding that some, possibly only a few, afferents bifurcate peripherally, actually innervating both somatic and visceral tissues. A more often discussed and experimentally supported theory is that afferents from visceral and somatic structures actually converge onto common spinal neurons. Activity from these neurons is transmitted rostrally and the message incorrectly interpreted by the brain as originating in the somatic instead of the visceral structures. Theoretically the convergent neurons could be localised supraspinally but experimental evidence is lacking.

A second phenomenon of importance for localisation of pain is projection of pain. An illustration may be the projection of the activity set up by stimulating the ulnar nerve at the elbow to the ring and little fingers. That a person will localise the sensation following stimulation of the peripheral nerve or nerve tract to the area for the normal origination of the receptors and afferents is believed to depend on a cortical mechanism, based on central somatotopic organisation of sensory input. Clinically, phantom pain is an illustration of the phenomenon—patients with distal nerve injury following amputation of a limb experience sensations and pain from the non-existing distal parts.

Spinal mechanisms in relation to secondary hyperalgesia or allodynia

The finding of primary hyperalgesia in a subject or patient with an injured or inflamed skin area has been discussed earlier. However, in the area surrounding the injury a secondary area of disturbed sensation develops, characterised by touch stimuli, activating Aβ-fibres and provoking painful sensations (secondary hyperalgesia or touch allodynia); (Fig. 1.6). Both primary and secondary hyperalgesia can be induced using mechanical, thermal or chemical stimuli. Following surgery the wound area is extremely sensitive to touch, leading to a significant problem of movement-related pain based on such hyperalgesia and allodynia. The mechanisms of secondary hyperalgesia or touch allodynia in this situation are considered to depend primarily on spinal cord mechanisms. Activity in primary nociceptive afferents from the injured area induces increased sensitivity in dorsal horn neurons, a central sensitisation. Besides increased facilitation of nociceptive transmission, the receptive field of dorsal horn neurons increases in size and changes response characteristics. Animal

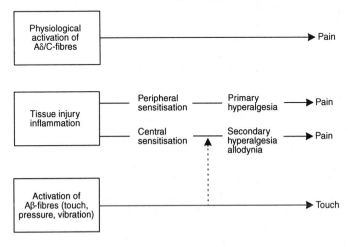

Fig 1.6 The importance of sensitisation for touch-evoked pain (allodynia) in clinical pain or pain due to pathology

15

research has shown that activity in C-fibres induces an enlargement of receptive fields in nociceptive-specific neurons, but it also permits the dorsal horn neurons to start to respond to non-noxious stimuli. One explanation of this change in response characteristics has been related to the activation of normally inefficient (subthreshold) synapses. It is documented in human volunteers that input in C-fibres is needed for initiating and developing secondary hyperalgesia or allodynia. A positive relation between the area of altered sensation and the activity in afferent C-fibres has been found in volunteers using experimental pain models, and in patients.

The exact mechanisms of these central changes have been related to a release of EAAs (aspartate and glutamate) and tachykinins from primary afferents and the activation of NMDA and non-NMDA-receptors as well as tachykinin-receptors on dorsal horn neurons. This leads to significant activation and longstanding increase in excitability of the neurons, providing a basis for the central sensitisation that leads to, for example, touch-evoked allodynia. Clinically it is interesting that ketamine, a drug normally used to induce general anaesthesia but known to possess analgesic properties in low doses, is a non-competitive NMDA antagonist. Ketamine has been found effective in reducing central sensitisation in human volunteers during experimentally induced pain when studying central summation, but also in patients suffering postoperative pain and in neuropathic pain.

Afferent pathways

After the first synapse in the dorsal horn, the second-order neuron transmits the activity to supraspinal areas via specific pathways. Most nociceptive fibres in the spinal cord project to brain regions via pathways in the ventrolateral white matter of the spinal cord, which are named according to their projecting areas (Fig. 1.7).

Pathways involved in pain signalling terminate in different areas in the brain. The spinothalamic tract is generally considered to be the most important pathway in pain transmission, which has been proved in several studies where this pathway has been lesioned. It projects directly to the ventroposterior lateral (VPL) nucleus in the thalamus, and is probably mainly responsible for the perception of well-localised pain sensations. The spinothalamic tract finally terminates in the somatosensory area of the cerebral cortex. The spinoreticular and spinomesencephalic tracts contact different nuclei in the brain stem before they reach the thalamus. At brain stem level the signal is transferred to different nuclei interacting with basic body functions such as breathing and circulation. Descending inhibitory pathways may also be activated, leading to a modulation of the nociceptive activity in the spinal cord.

16

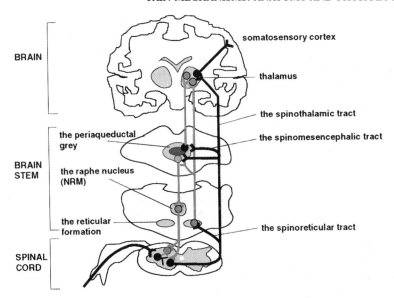

Fig 1.7   Ascending (black) and descending (grey) pathways of relevance for pain and its control

The spinoreticular tract is believed to be of importance for the affective component in pain perception. This tract contacts brain areas in the limbic system which is involved in emotional functions. Arousal may also be triggered by this pathway. The role of the spinomesencephalic tract is not well understood. It projects to a number of areas responsible for sensory-discriminatory functions, emotional responses, and descending inhibitory pathways.

Pathways located in the dorsal part of the spinal white matter are in general considered to convey non-painful sensory information. However, after ventrolateral cordotomy in pain syndromes, pain signalling in some cases reappeared after some months, suggesting dorsal pathways have a potential role in pain.

Thalamic neurons can be classified in the same manner as dorsal horn neurons, where there is one population of NS neurons and another, multireceptive, cell type, WDR neurons. This division is also useful for classifying neurons in the somatosensory cortex.

In line with the organisation in the spinal cord and the thalamic nucleus, the primary somatosensory cortex is somatotopically organised. As mentioned before, the sensory cortex is not the only region in the brain involved in pain perception. The frontal cortex is thought to be involved in the emotional part of the pain experience. Patients suffering from severe chronic pain, treated with neurosurgery to interrupt these paths, report that they can still perceive pain but they no longer describe it as unpleasant.

17

Endogenous pain-controlling mechanisms

Nociceptive activity can be modulated primarily at three levels: at the distal portion of the primary afferent, in the spinal cord, and in supraspinal areas (Fig. 1.8).

Peripheral opioid mechanisms

Since the nociceptive afferents through their peripheral branches can interact with surrounding tissues and cells, they become an obvious target for controlling nerve impulse activation and/or the release of proinflammatory peptides. Both animal and human data have recently been collected documenting a peripheral opioid control mechanism. Animal studies have shown that peripheral administration of opioids into the knee joint decreases the release of SP and CGRP from peptidergic C-fibres, probably

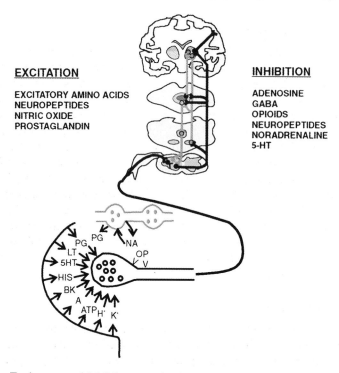

Fig 1.8   Excitatory and inhibitory mechanisms both in the peripheral and central nervous system. In the periphery, part of a postganglionic sympathetic efferent is depicted (grey) close to the nociceptive afferent. In the CNS, ascending tracts (black) and descending control (grey) are indicated with the corresponding excitatory and inhibitory neurotransmitters named at left and right hands, respectively.   A = adenosine;   ATP = adenosine   triphosphate;   BK = bradykinin; H^+ = hydrogen ions;   HIS = histamine; K^+ = potassium ions;   LT = leukotrienes; NA = noradrenaline; OP = opioid receptors; PG = prostaglandins; 5-HT = serotonin

due to an interaction with opioid receptors on afferent joint fibres. Later studies have shown that all three classes of opioid receptors (μ-, κ- and δ-) are present in peripheral tissues and that endogenous opioid peptides are produced by immunologically active cells such as monocytes and macrophages. It has therefore been proposed that during inflammation, endogenous opioids are released, binding to opioid receptors on afferents, resulting in decreased excitability and reduced release of peptides from the afferents. In patients undergoing knee joint surgery this hypothesis has been tested by local intra-articular injections of the opioid antagonist naloxone which resulted in increased pain, showing that an endogenous peripheral opioid control mechanism may have a pathophysiological role in pain and inflammation. Several clinical studies have documented significant analgesia in patients receiving intra-articular morphine for postoperative pain after knee joint surgery.

Segmental interaction

Nociceptive activity can be modulated at several levels. In 1965 Melzack and Wall presented their gate control for the modulation of pain within the nervous system. One important aspect of the theory was the proposal that activity in large myelinated afferents (sensitive to touch, pressure, and vibration) could result in the inhibition of nociceptive afferents or neurons activated by these afferents, through mechanisms of pre- and/or post-synaptic inhibition. A clinical spin-off from the theory was the introduction and development of transcutaneous electrical nerve stimulation (TENS) but also more elaborate forms such as dorsal column stimulation (DCS) for treatment of various painful conditions. Interestingly, afferent stimulation can also result in sympathetic inhibition and vasodilatation, which is of importance when treating ischaemic pain. The theory was conceptually important for introducing the notion of an early synaptic interaction within the nociceptive system, in fact already at the first synaptic area in the dorsal horn of the spinal cord.

Descending control

The fact that there exist centrifugal, efferent, control systems within the CNS has been known for more than 50 years through early anatomical and later pioneering electrophysiological studies. In the 1950s, experimental data were presented documenting corticofugal systems descending to the spinal cord and modulating somatosensory transmission. This aspect of central control was also discussed in the gate theory.

Descending inhibitory control of nociceptive transmission has been discussed over several decades, and interest grew when Reynolds (1969) showed that stimulation of discrete brain areas produced analgesia. Today it is well established that some brain stem areas make an important contribution to pain modulation. The periaqueductal grey (PAG) is probably the best studied area but the raphe nuclei (NRM) and the locus coeruleus are also key sites for pain inhibition. The most important projection for PAG neurons is NRM, where a majority of the neurons seem to be responsive to PAG stimulation. The PAG project to other nuclei such as the nucleus paragigantocellularis (PGi) and the pericoerular region, but these nuclei do not have the same impact on descending inhibition as the NRM nucleus does.

These brain stem areas can be activated by pathways arising in cortical or thalamic areas. This may explain why pain perception can be modulated by psychological stimuli such as hypnosis or stress. The descending inhibitory activity can also be set up by activity transmitted in ascending tracts, reaching these brain stem areas through collaterals. Thus, a negative feedback loop between activating nociceptive activity reaching brain stem areas resulting in increased descending activity feeding back into the dorsal horn of the spinal cord can decrease nociception and pain. One physiological significance of this system would be to provide the organism with a pain-controlling and regulating system specific for pain and activated only when needed. Animal data have shown that the system is activated during inflammation and pain. Whether the system is also tonically active is a matter for discussion. It is obviously of interest to find out the importance of the endogenous pain control systems in humans. One illustration is studies of patients suffering postoperative pain. Preoperatively the concentrations of endogenous opioids were determined in cerebrospinal fluid (CSF). Postoperatively the patients could self-administer opioids intravenously on demand, using patient-controlled analgesia (PCA). Interestingly, there was a negative correlation between preoperative CSF concentration of endogenous opioids and the postoperative need for opioid analgesics. A second factor of interest in understanding endogenous pain control is placebo phenomena, as studied in the postoperative setting for example. In patients subjected to surgery the opioid antagonist naloxone was administered postoperatively to patients first treated with placebo. Interestingly, part of the placebo response could be reversed, suggesting a role for endogenous opioids.

The transmitters involved in the descending control system at the spinal cord level are primarily 5-HT and noradrenaline (NA). The axons descend mainly in the dorsolateral funiculus to finally terminate in the dorsal horn at different spinal levels where they may act inhibitorily directly upon nociceptive neurons or by activating inhibitory interneurons. The action of local interneurons in the dorsal horn is in general considered to be mediated through that of endogenous opioid peptides or NA. More recent data, however, also emphasise cholinergic neurons as an important link.

Another interesting aspect of endogenous controls is that the fact that dorsal horn neurons activated by nociceptive afferents from one body area may also be inhibited by nociceptive activation from a different body area. The phenomenon that nociceptive activity can inhibit other spinal cord neurons than those directly activated by the afferents is called diffuse noxiously inhibitory controls (DNIC). A prerequisite for DNIC is an intact connection between spinal cord and brain stem areas such as PAG/NRM and a descending loop in the dorsolateral funiculus (DLF). In patients with spinal cord lesions DNIC is not present at a spinal level below the injury, demonstrating the need for intact ascending and descending pathways. One physiological function suggested for DNIC is to create a "contrast" in spinal outflow of nervous activity reaching supraspinal areas and resulting in increased pain intensity. Activity from an injured tissue would result in increased inhibition of nociceptive neurons innervating other areas, contrasting the primarily activated spinal cord neurons from the rest. The administration of opioids would then decrease DNIC, resulting in less contrast and correspondingly less pain or even analgesia. The administration of morphine to volunteers decreases DNIC under experimental conditions.

Pre-emptive analgesia—can pain be prevented?

During recent years the possibility of pre-empting pain following surgery has been intensively discussed. One starting point was the work by Wall, Woolf and collaborators documenting that brief activity in nociceptive C-fibres induced a long-lasting increase in the excitability of dorsal horn neurons. Interestingly, it was shown that central sensitisation was decreased more effectively if opioids were given before, as opposed to after, activating the afferents. Early clinical studies showed that administration of local anaesthetics/analgesics before surgery seemed to be a more efficacious way of reducing postoperative pain than starting after surgery when the patient first experienced pain. More recent studies have been less convincing regarding clinical significance.

There are at least three principal ways to address pre-emptive analgesia starting the analgesic treatment before surgery:

1 *To decrease the possibility of activation of nociceptive afferents.* During surgery tissue damage and inflammatory reactions lead to an activation of the nociceptive afferents through the release of various algogenic substances. Using clinically available drugs (NSAIDs, local anaesthetics), it is possible to interfere with some of these mechanisms.

2 *To reduce the possibility of activity in nociceptive afferents reaching spinal cord neurons.* It is obvious that prevention of activity in nociceptive afferents reaching the dorsal horn reduces central sensitisation. Clinically this is achieved using local anaesthetics to block nerve impulse propagation due to sodium-channel block.

3 *To reduce the possibility of nociceptive transmission within the CNS.* If activity

21

still reaches the CNS, premedication with adequate substances could decrease segmental and ascending transmission within the system. Clinically, opioids, α_2-agonists or NMDA antagonists would be one means of decreasing excitability in nociceptive neurons.

It is easy to understand the clinical interest in reducing postoperative pain by adequate preoperative treatment. Analysing the animal models used, it is obvious that treatment should not only start preoperatively but should continue through an essential part of the postoperative period, considering the continued activity in nociceptive afferents and the persisting source of central sensitisation.

Selected reading

Dickenson AH. Spinal pharmacology of pain. *Br J Anaesth* 1995;75:193–200.
Dray A. Inflammatory mediators of pain. *Br J Anaesth* 1995;75;125–31.
Fields HL. *Pain*. New York: McGraw-Hill, 1987.
Hökfelt T, Zhang X, Wiesenfeld-Hallin Z. Messenger plasticity in primary sensory neurons following axotomy and its functional implications. *TINS* 1994;1:22–30.
McMahon SB, Dmitrieva N, Koltzenburg M. Visceral pain. *Br J Anaesth* 1995;75:132–44.
Wall PD, Melzack R. *Textbook of pain*, 3rd edn. Edinburgh: Churchill Livingstone, 1994.
Woolf CJ. Somatic pain—pathogenesis and prevention. *Br J Anaesth* 1995;75:169–76.

2: Pharmacology of acute and chronic pain

ROBERT ATCHESON and DAVID J ROWBOTHAM

There are two principle reasons for the considerable advance in recent years in the pharmacological management of acute and chronic pain. Firstly, there is a greater and more widespread understanding of the pharmacology of drugs used in pain management. Secondly, the development of sophisticated, reliable and relatively inexpensive drug delivery systems, for example PCA and spinal drug administration. No new drug with superior efficacy and wide therapeutic index has been introduced recently. Rather, it has been better application of well-established drugs that have made significant contributions to pain management.

Opioid analgesics

The opioid analgesics are a diverse group of drugs possessing a number of similar structural, dynamic and kinetic characteristics. This section discusses mechanisms of opioid action and common pharmacokinetic and dynamic properties. Finally, the characteristics of individual drugs will be considered.

Although the terms "opioid" and "opiate" are often used interchangeably, they do have distinct definitions. An opioid is any drug acting at the opioid receptor. An opiate, for example morphine, codeine, papaverine, is a naturally occurring opioid derived from opium (from the Greek "opion", poppy juice). The term "narcotic" (from the Greek "narco", to be numb) is used also, but more commonly in a legal sense to indicate a drug of addition.

Mechanism of action

Opioids exert their pharmacological effect by acting as agonists at endogenous opioid receptors. There are three types of opioid receptors, μ (mu), δ (delta), and κ (kappa), and all three have been cloned. Their corresponding endogenous agonists are the endomorphins, enkephalins and dynorphins, respectively. Sub-receptors have been proposed, in particular μ_1 (analgesia) and μ_2 (respiratory depression). However, this is based on pharmacological experiments; as yet, no sub-receptor has been cloned and the search for a potent pure μ_1-agonist has been unsuccessful, despite the best efforts of the pharmaceutical industry over many years. A summary of the properties of each receptor type is given in Table 2.1.

In the CNS, the most important effects of opioid receptor activation are inhibition of excitatory neurotransmitter release from presynaptic terminals and hyperpolarisation of postsynaptic membranes decreasing the response of pain pathways to nociceptive stimuli. This may occur at spinal or supraspinal sites in the CNS. In the spinal cord, opioid receptors are found at the terminal zones of C-fibres, primarily in lamina I and the substantia gelatinosa. In the rat spinal cord, it has been reported that the relative density of μ-, δ-, and κ-receptors is 70%, 24% and 6%, respectively. Direct application of μ-agonists to the spinal cord produces analgesia but no loss of other sensation. More than 70% of the μ-receptors are on the afferent

Table 2.1 Several drugs in this table are restricted to the laboratory but are important because they have helped to characterise the various pharmacological receptor subtypes. Naloxone is an antagonist at all three receptors

	Receptor		
	μ	δ	κ
Endogenous ligand	β-Endomorphin	Enkephalin	Dynorphin
Exogenous agonist	Morphine, fentanyl, DAMGO	DPDPE DSLET	Enadoline Pentazocine
Antagonist	Naloxonazine, CTOP	Naltrindole	NorBNI
Pharmacological subtypes	1,2,3	1,2	1,2,3
K^+-channel conductance	Increases	Increases	Increases
Adenyl cyclase	Inhibits	Inhibits	Inhibits
Voltage-dependent Ca^{2+} channels	Inactivates	Inactivates	Inactivates
Function	Analgesia Respiratory depression Constipation	Analgesia ? Respiratory depression	Analgesia Diuresis Dysphoria ? Respiratory depression

CTOP = H-D-Phe-Cys-Tyr-D-Trp-Orn-Thr-Pen-Thr-NH$_2$; DAMGO = [D-Ala^2, Me Phe^4, gly-Col)^5]enkephalin; DPDPE = [D-Pen^{2,5}]enkephalin; DSLET = [D-Ser^2, Leu^5]enkephalin-Thr^6; NorBNI = norbinal torphimine.

terminals. Stimulation of the presynaptic μ- and δ-receptors is associated with hyperpolarisation of the terminal and reduced neurotransmitter release. Some opioid receptors are situated on the postsynaptic membrane and the precise mechanism for reduction in nociception on stimulation of these receptors is not clear. Direct application of selective δ- and, to a lesser extent, κ-agonists results in spinal analgesia also.

There are multiple supraspinal sites involved in pain modulation, in particular, the PAG and NRM in the brain stem. Activation increases tone in descending monoamine pathways which interact with pain transmission in the spinal cord. Spinal and supraspinal analgesia are synergistic and systemically applied opioids exert effects at both sites.

At a cellular level, opioid receptor activation has been shown to be associated with increased potassium-channel conductance, inhibition of adenyl cyclase and inactivation of voltage-dependent calcium channels (Table 2.1).

Potency and efficacy

In order to understand the pharmacology of opioids, and indeed all drugs, it is important to understand the relation between potency and efficacy. These terms are specific pharmacological definitions and their use is often confused. Fig. 2.1 shows the log dose–response curve of a typical μ-agonist. A typical sigmoid curve is displayed and the potency of drug A is

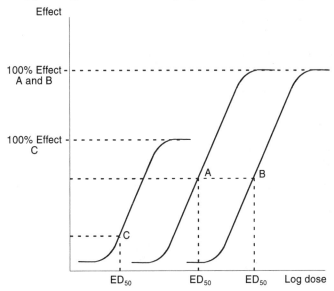

Fig 2.1　Log dose–response curve of typical μ-agonists. Drugs A and B have similar efficacies, but drug A is more potent than B, i.e. ED_{50} of A<B. Drug C has less efficacy than A and B but is more potent

shown by the ED_{50}—the dose required to produce 50% of the maximum response. The maximum response is the efficacy. Drug B is a similar drug but because the dose response is shifted to the right the ED_{50} and therefore potency is less than drug A. However, they have the same efficacy (magnitude of 100% response). Drug C is a typical partial agonist. Its maximum effect is about 50% of drugs A and C and therefore its efficacy is less. However, in this particular case, its potency is greater than drug A and B because the dose–response curve is to the left of the others and the ED_{50} is less. This could be the dose response of buprenorphine (very potent but low efficacy).

Classification of opioids

According to tradition, commonly used opioids have been divided into strong, intermediate and weak, according to their perceived analgesic properties. However, this division is misleading and potentially hazardous, as it may imply that "weak" opioids are safer. The most widely used "weak" opioid is codeine, often used in combination with paracetamol or aspirin. Its "weakness" simply reflects its relatively low potency compared with morphine. At doses equipotent to morphine, it has a similar propensity for important side-effects such as respiratory depression.

The term "intermediate" opioid is often applied to either partial μ-agonists which have a limited efficacy at the μ-receptor, or mixed agonist-antagonists, i.e. an agonist at one opioid receptor type and antagonist at another. Their limited popularity reflects poor efficacy compared with "strong" opioids and a relatively high incidence of opioid side-effects, especially nausea and vomiting. The term "strong" opioid is applied to relatively potent pure opioid agonists, for example morphine, pethidine, fentanyl, alfentanil, sufentanil, etc.

Structurally, opioids may be divided into three groups:

1 The morphinans, e.g. morphine
2 4-Phenylpiperidines, e.g. pethidine, fentanyl
3 3,3-Diphenylpropylamines, e.g. methadone, dextropropoxyphene.

The three types are complex polycyclic structures and quite closely related. In fact, the phenylpiperidines and diphenylpropylamines are structurally derived from the morphinans. With the advent of remifentanil, a new structural class can be included—opioids with ester linkages.

Pharmacokinetics

The simple pharmacokinetic values for the commonly used opioids are given in Table 2.2. The speed of onset of an intravenous bolus of an opioid is dependent on the rate of diffusion from the capillary to the receptor of the non-ionised, non-protein-bound fraction of the drug. The rate of diffusion depends on lipid solubility and the concentration gradient. Morphine has a

Table 2.2 Typical pharmacokinetics of some commonly used opioids. Average data are presented; it should be remembered that there is considerable interpatient variability

	Volume of distribution (litre/kg)	Clearance (ml/min/kg)	Elimination half-life (h)
Morphine	3·5	15	3
Codeine	2·6	11	2·9
Methadone	3·8	1·4	35
Oxycodone	2·6	9·7	3·7
Hydromorphone	4·1	22	3·1
Pentazocine	7·1	17	4·6
Nalbuphine	3·8	22	2·3
Pethidine	4·0	12	4
Alfentanil	0·8	6	1·6
Fentanyl	4·0	13	3·5
Sufentanil	1·7	12·7	2·7

relatively slow onset for two reasons: firstly, it has a high pK_a (8.0), therefore only a small fraction is unionised in the plasma; secondly, because of its two polar hydroxyl groups, it is relatively hydrophilic. In contrast, alfentanil has a rapid onset because it has a low pK_a and is relatively lipophilic.

At steady-state plasma concentrations, the effective duration depends upon the elimination half-life, which itself depends upon the volume of distribution and the drug clearance. Methadone has a long elimination half-life allowing once or twice daily administration, which gives it a distinct clinical advantage over other opioids. In contrast, morphine (unless as a slow release preparation) must be given approximately four hourly. In general, opioids have a large volume of distribution (see Table 2.2). The relatively small volume of distribution of alfentanil accounts for its short half-life.

Systemic activity following oral administration is dependent on first pass metabolism, which is relatively high for most opioids and for some approaches 100%, for example fentanyl. Exceptions are methadone, oxycodone and, to a lesser extent, codeine (Table 2.3).

Table 2.3 Typical oral bioavailabilities of some commonly used opioids

	Bioavailability (%)
Morphine	25
Codeine	50
Methadone	92
Oxycodone	60
Pethidine	52
Hydromorphone	50
Pentazocine	47
Nalbuphine	16

27

Although a knowledge of individual drug pharmacokinetics allows a more rational approach to therapy, large differences in pharmacokinetics occur between patients. Consequently, in order to produce good analgesia with minimal side-effects, it must be appreciated that there are large and unpredictable variations in constant infusion rates, times to peak concentration after intramuscular injection and dosage of all methods of administration. Similar pharmacokinetic differences occur with spinally administered opioids, both intrathecal or epidural. It is important to remember that published pharmacokinetic data for individual drugs are means of a wide distribution. Dose should always be titrated to effect when administering opioids.

Pharmacodynamics

Most opioids have a narrow therapeutic index. Furthermore, when they have been measured, effective plasma concentrations vary considerably. Therefore, there are pharmacodynamic, as well as pharmacokinetic reasons why opioids must be titrated to effect in each individual.

Central nervous system

The inhibitory effects of opioids in the CNS contribute towards analgesia, sedation and respiratory depression. However, opioids exhibit excitatory mechanisms which account for nausea and vomiting (see below) and meiosis (indirect stimulation of the Edinger–Westphal nucleus of the third cranial nerve). The euphoric effects of opioids often contribute to the analgesic effect. Dysphoria is more commonly seen with large doses, and is often exacerbated by general debility, constipation, and poor pain control. More subtle side-effects such as day-time somnolence, lethargy, and poor concentration are common complaints with prolonged administration.

Respiration

Respiratory depression occurs with all commonly used opioids and arises from a direct depression of brain stem respiratory centres. Respiratory rate and tidal volume are reduced and the respiratory pattern may become irregular, with periods of apnoea, particularly when the patient is asleep. There is a shift to the right of the carbon dioxide response curve and the slope is decreased. The respiratory response to hypoxia is impaired also, an important consideration in the postoperative period.

Initially, a profound reduction in ventilation is not necessarily associated with loss of consciousness and patients will breathe when instructed to do so. Respiratory depression is not often associated with chronic use but may become a problem if pain is relieved suddenly with a regional technique. Delayed respiratory depression has been reported after spinal administration. This is a particular problem with the less lipid soluble opioids, for example morphine. There are no differences in the potential for respiratory depression between opioids at equianalgesic doses.

Gastrointestinal and urological systems

Opioids induce nausea and vomiting by activation of the chemoreceptor trigger zone in the area postrema of the medulla and possibly by its gastrointestinal effects. Nausea is enhanced by vestibular stimulation, for example walking, moving in bed. Tolerance to nausea may develop rapidly.

Opioids decrease gastric motility and gastric emptying time. Small and large bowel tone is increased and propulsive contractions are reduced. Delayed transit time through the bowel increases water absorption and faecal desiccation, further contributing to constipation. This is enhanced also by reduced reflex response to rectal distension. These effects are mediated through opioid receptors in the bowel wall, although central mechanisms may contribute.

Opioids constrict the sphincter of Oddi, increasing pressure within the biliary tract. Urinary retention is common although tolerance develops rapidly. Increased tone in the detrusor and external sphincter of the bladder and inhibition of the voiding reflex are the likely causes.

Cardiovascular system

Most opioids reduce sympathetic tone and may cause hypotension, particularly in patients dependent on high sympathetic tone, the elderly and patients with poor cardiac function. Bradycardia is more common than tachycardia, except for pethidine; this may reflect pethidine's structural similarity to atropine. Like most opioid-induced side-effects, cardiovascular instability is far more frequent after parenteral administration, in association with high peak and rapidly changing plasma concentrations. Many workers have described the relative cardiovascular stability of the newer opioids in cardiac surgery, where doses are much higher. These data are not relevant to acute or chronic pain.

Skin and pruritus

Many opioids, for example morphine and pethidine, induce histamine release from mast cells in a dose-dependent manner. This usually manifests itself as flushing, usually in the upper half of the body, mild to moderate hypotension and pruritus. This is a direct interaction and not mediated via opioid receptors and therefore not reversed with naloxone. The incidence and severity are reduced by the use of small increments rather than a single large bolus. In contrast, pruritus following spinal administration of opioids, which may occur with drugs that do not cause pruritus following parenteral injection, may be reversed with naloxone, implying an opioid receptor mediated mechanism.

Tolerance, dependence, and addiction

These terms are often used in discussion during the management of patients with opioids; they have precise definitions and are often confused.

Tolerance is a phenomena where an increasing dose of drug is required for a given effect. It may be receptor mediated, for example opioids, or metabolically mediated, for example hepatic enzyme induction. Dependence is a state in which an abstinence syndrome may occur following either abrupt withdrawal of the drug, a large dose reduction, or the administration of an antagonist. Addiction is a behavioural pattern of drug use, characterised by compulsive self-administration on a continuous or periodic basis in order to experience its psychic effects and sometimes to avoid discomfort of its absence, often securing supply by deceptive or illegal means.

Although tolerance to opioids may be demonstrated within a few days, it has little clinical relevance in most patients on chronic opioid therapy, who are usually suffering from cancer. Tolerance to adverse effects occurs more rapidly than to analgesia, with the exception of constipation. Increased dose requirements may imply disease progression rather than tolerance *per se*. However, rapid dose reduction, for example following the introduction of spinal opioids, may precipitate a withdrawal reaction because opioids induce a state of physical dependence. Drug addiction is extremely rare in cancer patients with no history of drug abuse.

When used for acute pain, addiction is also extremely rare. However, tolerance and dependence may occur during prolonged administration. This should not inhibit the use of opioids for the relief of pain in the postoperative period. It is often stated that the chances of becoming addicted to opioids are far greater in those administering the drug than those receiving it.

Individual opioids

Equianalgesic doses of some commonly used opioids are shown in Table 2.4

Morphine

Morphine (from Morpheus, Greek god of dreams) is the parent molecule of the morphinans and the standard by which other opioids are compared. It was first isolated from opium in 1806 and synthesised in 1952. Raw opium (extract of the poppy *Papaver somniferum*) remains the cheapest source of medicinal morphine and consists of over 25 alkaloids, of which morphine constitutes 9–17%. Morphine and morphine-like drugs can be given in equianalgesic doses since they exhibit similar efficacy at the receptor, although potency varies greatly. Oral bioavailability of morphine is approximately 25% and rectal bioavailability is similar. Metabolism occurs through conjugation with glucuronic acid in the liver, producing morphine-6-glucuronide (M6G) and morphine-3-glucuronide (M3G) which are excreted in urine and accumulate in renal impairment. A secondary pathway involves demethylation to produce normorphine. M6G is an active metabolite with a greater potency than morphine. M3G is inactive; it has even been suggested that it has an antagonist-like effect but this is still controversial and not generally accepted. There is no change in the pharmacokinetics of morphine when used for long term treatment in cancer patients, even with a 10–20 fold increase in dose.

Papaveretum is a mixture of opium alkaloids, the principle constituents being morphine (50%), codeine, papaverine, and noscapine. Noscapine may be teratogenic and is no longer a component of commercially available papaveretum in the UK.

Codeine

Codeine (3-methoxy morphine) has an oral bioavailability of approximately 50% and a half-life of 2–4 hours. It is metabolised in the liver mainly by glucuronidation but also by N-demethylation (norcodeine) and O-demethylation (morphine). Codeine has a low affinity for opioid receptors and it is likely that its analgesic efficacy is due to conversion to morphine (about 10%). Metabolism to morphine is by the genetically polymorphic CYP2D6 enzyme; this enzyme is not present in some individuals, for example 7% of the white population. Therefore, a small but

Table 2.4 Equianalgesic doses of some commonly used opioids

Drug and route	Equianalgesic dose (mg)	Duration (h)
Morphine		
IM	10	3–5
PO	30–60	
Codeine		
IM	120	3–6
PO	200	
Hydromorphone		
IM	1·5	3–6
PO	3·0	
Methadone		
IM	8–10	3–4 (single dose)
PO	10	6–24 (steady state)
Pethidine		
IM	75–100	2–3
PO	200	
Fentanyl		
IV	100 μg	0·75–1
Buprenorphin		
IM	0·3–0·6	8–10
SL	0·4–0·8	

IM = intramuscular; IV = intravenous; PO = oral; SL = sublingual.

significant number of patients are unlikely to derive any benefit from codeine. Several drugs (e.g. tricyclic antidepressants) inhibit this enzyme and may reduce the analgesic efficacy of codeine. Codeine is often prescribed in combination with paracetamol or aspirin.

Diamorphine

Diamorphine (3,6-diacetyl morphine, or heroin) is a semisynthetic opioid with a very high clearance because of its rapid conversion to 6-monoacetyl morphine (6-MAM), chiefly in the liver. 6-MAM is a potent opioid analgesic, and, in addition, is metabolised to morphine. Despite the commonly held belief that diamorphine has more pronounced euphoric properties with less nausea and vomiting, there are no significant pharmacodynamic differences between morphine and diamorphine at equianalgesic doses. However, when administered spinally, its high lipid solubility ensures a more rapid onset than morphine.

Hydromorphone

Hydromorphone is a semisynthetic opioid which is about six times more potent than morphine, with a similar duration of action but greater bioavailability (see Table 2.3). It is relatively hydrophilic and excreted primarily as the 3-glucuronide; little or no 6-glucuronide is produced. It may be better tolerated than morphine by some patients.

Methadone

Methadone is a synthetic opioid and may cause less euphoria and sedation. It has a high oral bioavailability (see Table 2.3) and undergoes hepatic and renal clearance. Single dosage produces a similar quality and duration of analgesia to the same dose of morphine because the duration of action under these circumstances is limited by the redistribution half-life. However, the elimination half-life of methadone is 20–45 hours (see Table 2.2) and significant accumulation occurs. It may take up to 10 days to reach steady-state plasma concentration during oral administration. Consequently, a once daily dosage is possible when steady state has been reached. A regimen of 10 mg at 0, 6, 12 and 24 hours, followed by 10 mg on day 3, has been suggested as initial therapy. Because it may be given on a once daily regimen, it is useful not only for chronic pain but also in drug rehabilitation programmes. Its efficacy in cancer pain is well proved.

Pethidine

Pethidine (meperidine) was first synthesised in 1939 in an attempt to develop an atropine substitute. It has an oral bioavailability of approximately 50% and is metabolised by hydrolysis to inactive compounds and by N-demethylation to norpethidine. The latter may accumulate with repeated dosing and in high concentrations causes central excitation and convulsions. Pethidine has a shorter duration of action than morphine (2–3 hours) and, coupled with a risk of norpethidine accumulation, is unsuitable for repeated administration. Pethidine is contraindicated in patients taking monoamine oxidase inhibitors.

Because of its structural similarity to atropine, it has an anticholinergic effect. It also has a membrane stabilising effect and has been used as a local anaesthetic.

Fentanyl and derivatives

Fentanyl was introduced in the early 1960s and is about 100 times more potent than morphine. Related drugs, in increasing potency, are alfentanil, sufentanil, and lofentanil.

Fentanyl has a high hepatic clearance and is not available as an oral preparation. It is metabolised to inactive compounds, initially by N-dealkylation to norfentanyl, which are excreted in urine. It may be used in PCA as an alternative to morphine or pethidine, as an infusion or epidurally, often in combination with a local anaesthetic as a continuous infusion.

Fentanyl has a high lipid solubility which makes it suitable for transdermal administration. Self-adhesive fentanyl patches are available which release the drug at a constant rate (25, 50, 75, and 100 μg/h). The patches last 72 hours and changes in dose may take 24 hours to have full effect. Fentanyl patches may be an effective substitute for morphine in cancer pain when side-effects from morphine become intolerable. It is unsuitable for postoperative pain relief. Fentanyl has a relatively long eliminaton half-life and tends to form significant depots of drug in the skin. This explains the prolonged action of the patch after removal.

Remifentanil is a new potent opioid with an ester linkage in its structure. It is metabolised by non-specific esterases and therefore has a short and predictable half-life (10–20 minutes). Its role in the management of pain is yet to be evaluated.

Tramadol

Tramadol is a centrally acting analgesic with relatively weak μ-opioid receptor activity. However, it also inhibits monoamine reuptake. It is a mixture of two stereoisomers, and since each isomer exerts its main effect through different mechanisms, the combination may be synergistic. It has a potency similar to codeine and an efficacy similar to that of morphine has been claimed, but many practitioners would dispute this. The advantages over traditional opioids are absence of tolerance and addiction and minimum respiratory depression. However, it may cause vomiting, sedation, dry mouth, and headache.

Partial agonists

The partial agonists have limited efficacy at the μ-receptor, and once reached, increasing the dose does not increase analgesia. The advantage of partial agonists is a ceiling effect on respiratory depression (but dangerous respiratory depression may occur), less abuse potential than morphine, and less psychomimetic side-effects than the agonist-antagonists.

Buprenorphine

Buprenorphine is a partial μ-agonist that is approximately 30 times more potent than morphine. It is characterised by a high receptor affinity and slow receptor association and dissociation. Thus, peak effect may take 3 hours with a duration of action of 10 hours. If respiratory depression does occur, it may be difficult to reverse with naloxone alone because of the receptor kinetics.

Agonist-antagonists

The analgesic efficacy of the agonist-antagonists arises most commonly from κ-receptor activation, with antagonism at the μ-receptor, a feature noticeable in the presence of a μ-agonist such as morphine. Like the partial agonists, they can precipitate withdrawal symptoms in patients tolerant to morphine. Their advantages are similar to those of partial agonists; a ceiling effect on respiratory depression and limited abuse potential. However, dysphoria and nausea are common and this, along with reduced efficacy, limit their use. Drugs in this class include pentazocine, butorphanol, and nalbuphine.

Intrathecal and epidural administration of opioids

The spinal route has become more popular in recent years because it provides intense analgesia. This applies to acute pain in the opioid naive patient and to cancer patients with poorly controlled pain on high doses of opioids. The epidural route is more popular than the intrathecal route because of an intact dura protecting the cord from infection.

Factors affecting the pharmacokinetics of spinal opioids are similar to systemic injection. The speed of onset is determined mainly by the pK_a, the lipid solubility of the non-ionised fraction, and the concentration gradient. In particular, the more lipid soluble drugs (e.g. pethidine, fentanyl) have a more rapid onset but shorter duration compared with morphine. Less than 5% of an epidural dose of morphine crosses the dura but CSF concentrations are still approximately a 100-fold greater compared with intramuscular injection. Following either intrathecal or epidural injection, peak plasma concentrations occur within 10 minutes and may be sufficiently high to contribute to analgesia within the first hour, especially with lipid soluble drugs injected epidurally. This reflects uptake into either

Table 2.5 Suggested dose administration conversion table for morphine

Route	Dose ratio
Oral→intramuscular	3:1
Intramuscular→epidural	10:1
Epidural→intrathecal	10:1

epidural or cord vasculature. Following epidural injection, morphine crosses the dura slowly (absorption half-life 22 minutes), and maximum CSF concentrations after epidural administration occur at about 60–90 minutes. In contrast, pethidine crosses the dura at four times the rate of morphine but also declines four times quicker. After epidural injection, access to the CSF probably occurs via protrusions of arachnoid mater around nerve roots. After intrathecal injection, CSF opioid concentrations decline rapidly in the first 15 minutes and then more slowly; for example, morphine and pethidine have half-lives of 90 and 70 minutes, respectively. A low lipid solubility increases the possibility of rostral spread and delayed respiratory depression.

Analgesia following spinal morphine lasts about 12–24 hours but delayed respiratory depression may occur up to 24 hours after administration. However, respiratory depression is very unlikely in patients who are not opioid naive. Profound nausea and vomiting may occur, as may pruritus, although tolerance to both develop rapidly. If opioids are to be used spinally, they must be preservative free.

When converting from one method of morphine administration to another in patients with chronic pain, the choice of dose is an important consideration. A suitable conversion regimen for morphine has been suggested and is shown in Table 2.5.

Non-steroidal anti-inflammatory drugs and paracetamol (acetaminophen)

Mechanism of action

Tissue damage and inflammation lead to activation of prostaglandins, which stimulates peripheral nociceptors and sensitises them to other inflammatory mediators such as bradykinin. NSAIDs inhibit prostaglandin synthesis from arachidonic acid by inhibiting COX (Fig. 2.2). This accounts for the analgesic, antiplatelet, antipyretic, and anti-inflammatory effects. However, there is some evidence that analgesia may be mediated also by a central mechanism of action. For example, NSAIDs have been shown to reduce the spinal thalamic response to peripheral nociceptor stimulation. Furthermore, analgesic and anti-inflammatory potency are not always related. For example, azopropazone, diflunisal, and naproxen are effective analgesics but are weak inhibitors of prostaglandin synthesis. This may suggest that at least some of the analgesic action of these drugs is not related to prostaglandins.

NSAIDs demonstrate a ceiling effect for analgesia; further dose escalation increases adverse effects only. Differences in efficacy and side-effects between drugs may reflect variability against COX. In addition, pharmacokinetic differences contribute to significant interpatient variability in response.

There are two distinct types of COX enzyme, COX-1 and COX-2. COX-1 is produced under normal conditions and is present in healthy cells. It is important in the regulation of prostaglandin synthesis in the gastric mucosa and renal vascular bed. Inhibition of this enzyme is responsible for the gastrointestinal and renal side-effects of NSAIDs. During inflammation,

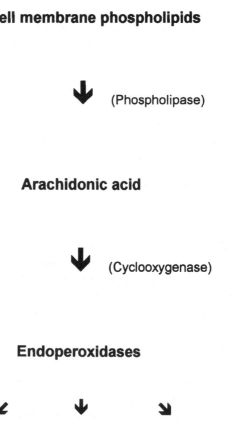

Cell membrane phospholipids

⬇ (Phospholipase)

Arachidonic acid

⬇ (Cyclooxygenase)

Endoperoxidases

↙ ⬇ ↘

Thromboxane   Prostaglandins   Prostacyclins

Fig 2.2   NSAIDs inhibit cyclooxygenase

endothelial cells, fibroblasts, and macrophages produce COX-2. It is likely that the relative inhibition of these two isoenzymes will be related to the likelihood of side-effects. Consequently, COX-2-specific NSAIDs are undergoing clinical trials at present with the hope of demonstrating good analgesia with few side-effects. The results of these trials are awaited with interest.

Paracetamol (acetaminophen) has analgesic and antipyretic properties similar to aspirin, but has virtually no anti-inflammatory activity. It is considered at the end of this section.

Pharmacokinetics

Absorption

NSAIDs are rapidly and almost completely absorbed from the upper small intestine and, to a lesser extent, from the stomach. Peak plasma concentrations are reached usually within 2 hours, but this is delayed and reduced if taken with food. Total absorption is unchanged.

Distribution

NSAIDs are highly bound (often >95%) to plasma protein and may displace other highly bound drugs, for example oral hypoglycaemics, anticonvulsants, warfarin, and sulphonamides. NSAIDs have a low apparent volume of distribution and most have short half-lives (2–3 hours). Drugs with long half-lives, for example naproxen and piroxicam, may be given once daily, although this advantage may extend to the remaining drugs through slow release formulations.

Elimination

Most NSAIDs undergo biotransformation and conjugation, followed by renal excretion. Only a very small fraction of the drug is excreted unchanged in the urine. Piroxicam plasma concentrations may show multiple peaks as a result of enterohepatic circulation. Most NSAIDs have inactive metabolites but some produce active metabolites, for example fenbufen, meclofenamic acid, nabumetone, phenylbutazone, and sulindac.

Side-effects

Gastrointestinal tract

Gastric mucosal damage is relatively common with all NSAIDs because of the inhibition of gastric mucus production. Nausea, vomiting, and epigastric pain are common, but dyspepsia does not predict severe gastric mucosal damage nor intestinal blood loss. The risk of gastrointestinal side-effects increases with age, smoking, high dosage, alcohol, anticoagulants (warfarin and heparin, including twice daily subcutaneous injections), and corticosteroids. Suppositories are not associated with a lower incidence of gastrointestinal side-effects. The use of H_2-antagonists or prostaglandin analogues, such as misoprostol, may reduce the incidence of side-effects.

Haematological

NSAIDs inhibit the formation of thromboxane A_2 and therefore platelet aggregation. Most NSAIDs exert their action on platelet function only when they are present in the circulation, but aspirin inhibits the enzyme irreversibly and so has a more prolonged effect on platelet aggregation which lasts 4–8 days. Increased bleeding times are associated with NSAID intake and increased blood loss after surgery has been reported. Rarely, blood dyscrasias may occur, such as thrombocytopenia and agranulocytosis.

Renal

Inhibition of prostaglandins which promote vasodilatation may cause acute, renal insufficiency. The risk is increased in patients with pre-existing reduced renal perfusion, for example hypovolaemia, heart failure, diuretic therapy, elderly. This is of particular importance when NSAIDs are used for postoperative analgesia. In addition, NSAIDs may cause allergic interstitial nephritis, nephrotic syndrome, and tubular dysfunction.

Drug interactions

Pharmacokinetic or pharmacodynamic effects of NSAIDs may produce a number of significant drug interactions. NSAIDs are strongly albumin bound and compete with other acidic drugs for albumin binding sites. Interactions causing NSAID displacement increase clearance but do not alter the free-fraction. Consequently, increased therapeutic or toxic effects are not normally seen.

Warfarin may be displaced by a NSAID and combined with the antiplatelet effects there may be potentiation of bleeding. Close monitoring of coagulation is essential on introduction or removal of NSAID treatment. Most NSAIDs reduce lithium clearance and increase plasma lithium concentrations. Azapropazone and others of the pyrazole group of NSAIDs have exacerbated the hypoglycaemic effect of tolbutamide. Ibuprofen, diclofenac, naproxen, and sulindac have no effect.

The pyrazole group will also increase the likelihood of phenytoin toxicity (albumin displacement and impairment of metabolism). Although other NSAIDs displace phenytoin from albumin, there is little effect on free drug, and therefore toxicity, unless hepatic clearance is saturated. Severe adverse effects have been reported with high dose methotrexate and this may be the result of competition for renal tubular elimination. Other interactions as a result of renal impairment are possible.

NSAIDs may reduce the effectiveness of any class of antihypertensive therapy. It is likely that NSAIDs have an effect on water and salt retention via a renal mechanism. Similarly, they may affect adversely any cardiac failure therapy. Hyperkalaemia may result if given with angiotensin-converting enzyme (ACE) inhibitors or potassium sparing diuretics. Antihypertensive or cardiac failure treatment may also increase the chances of adverse renal effects of NSAIDs themselves.

Individual NSAIDs

It is not possible to describe in any detail the specific pharmacology for all NSAIDs as there are numerous ones available world-wide; the following is a summary of important general points and those specific to commonly used drugs.

Salicylates

Aspirin (acetysalicylic acid) remains one of the most widely used analgesics. It is hydrolysed rapidly to salicylic acid, which has a plasma half-life of 2–3 hours. At low doses (300–600 mg) it is an analgesic and well tolerated, but in high doses needed for its anti-inflammatory effect over 50% of patients will suffer adverse effects, mainly gastrointestinal. The plasma half-life of salicylic acid is dose dependent (3–30 hours) because of rate-limiting hepatic conjugation. The risk of dyspepsia, but not gastro-intestinal blood loss, is reduced with enteric-coated preparations. Aspirin is contraindicated in children because of the association with Reye's syndrome.

Diflunisal (difluorophenyl derivative of salicylic acid) is more potent, has a longer duration, and is better tolerated than aspirin (no tinnitus, less gastrointestinal and platelet effects). It is not metabolised to salicylic acid *in vitro*.

Proprionic acids

These drugs are used very widely and are better tolerated than aspirin. Examples of this class include ibuprofen, naproxen, fenoprofen, and ketoprofen. There are few significant differences between the many drugs of this class. The use of a prodrug (fenbufen), in an attempt to reduce side-effects, has proved unsuccessful.

Indomethacin and sulindac

Indomethacin is a methylated indole derivative introduced in 1963. It has a high incidence of adverse effects (30–50%), particularly gastrointestinal. Sulindac is a derivative of indomethacin and it is likely that most of its activity is due to the sulphide metabolite. It appears to have less effect on renal function than other NSAIDs but should still be used with caution in renal impairment.

Diclofenac

Diclofenac is a phenylacetic acid derivative. It is absorbed rapidly but its bioavailability is only about 50% because of the first-pass effect. It has similar efficacy and adverse effects as proprionic acid derivatives.

Others

Nabumetone is a prodrug whose active metabolite (6-methoxy-2-naph-thylacetic acid) has a long elimination half-life, allowing once daily dosing. Piroxicam has a long half-life also (approximately 50 hours).

Which NSAID?

As the relative efficacy of NSAIDs is unclear the choice of drug is often influenced by the likelihood of side-effects. The suggestion that sulindac may be safer in renal impairment has been mentioned already. The Committee on the Safety of Medicines in the UK published the conclusions based on several studies and spontaneous reports. The risk of adverse events was high with azapropazone, moderate with diclofenac, ketoprofen, indomethacin, naproxen, and piroxicam, and low with ibuprofen.

Contraindications and precautions

NSAIDs are contraindicated in patients with a history of peptic ulcer disease. Extreme caution should be exercised with asthma and renal impairment, and patients at risk from bleeding. Aspirin may cause an acute and potentially life-threatening hypersensitivity reaction, similar to anaphylaxis, and cross-reactivity with other NSAIDs may occur. NSAIDs may cross the placenta and should be avoided during pregnancy and lactation.

Paracetamol (acetaminophen)

Paracetamol, the active derivative of phenacetin, has been widely used since the mid 1950s as an analgesic and antipyretic agent. Its mechanism of action is still unclear but it may selectively inhibit brain prostaglandin synthesis. It has very little activity against peripheral COX. Consequently, it has no anti-inflammatory activity and does not cause gastric ulceration and bleeding.

It is rapidly and almost completely absorbed from the small bowel and reaches peak plasma concentrations within 1 hour. It has a plasma half-life of 2–3 hours and plasma binding is variable (20–50%). It is metabolised in the liver, chiefly by conjugation with glucuronic and sulphuric acids, and the products excreted in urine. In recommended therapeutic doses, paracetamol is well tolerated with the occasional skin rash and hypersensitivity reaction. Cross hypersensitivity with aspirin is rare.

In large doses, usually after intentional overdose, paracetamol may cause potentially fatal hepatic necrosis. Normally, a small fraction of paracetamol undergoes metabolism via the cytochrome P-450 hepatic enzyme system, forming a highly reactive metabolite (N-acetyl-benzoquinoneimine). This metabolite reacts with the sulphydryl groups in glutathione and becomes non-toxic. It is the depletion of glutathione in paracetamol overdose that is responsible for the accumulation of the toxic metabolite and hepatic necrosis. Hepatotoxicity may occur after a single dose of 10–15 g, or even less with pre-existing liver disease.

The efficacy of paracetamol is often underestimated, particularly when used in combination with other analgesics.

Local anaesthetics

Mechanism of action

The function of neuronal cells is dependent on electrical excitability which generates action potentials. The resting membrane potential is approximately -70 mV, with the inside of the cell membrane negatively charged with respect to the outside. This is achieved by the action of the sodium-potassium ATPase pump which pumps sodium ions out of and potassium ions into the cell. At rest, the cell membrane is relatively permeable to potassium but impermeable to sodium. Excitation results in marked changes in ion permeability and therefore transmembrane potential. Following electrical stimulation, sodium channels open and become highly permeable. Sodium enters the cell rapidly, and the membrane potential changes from a threshold of approximately -50 mV to $+40$ mV. At the peak of the action potential, sodium channels close and become inactive. This initiates the repolarisation phase, which is largely attributed to an increase in potassium conductance and efflux from the cell. This accounts for a period of hyperpolarisation which precedes a return to the normal resting state. The absolute changes in ion concentrations are small since the duration of the action potential is only about 1 millisecond.

The primary effect of local anaesthetics is a decrease in the rate and magnitude of depolarisation because they interfere with sodium conductance. The sodium channel exists in one of three states: resting and closed; open and permeable during depolarisation; and inactive and closed immediately after depolarisation (absolute refractory period). Local anaesthetics bind to the channel with high affinity in the open and inactive states, but with low affinity in the resting state. This accounts for frequency-dependent blockade, in which onset of block is reduced with an increase in frequency of nerve stimulation. However, this characteristic is not seen with uncharged lipophilic drugs such as benzocaine. Therefore, it has been postulated that local anaesthetics may reach their receptor site in the sodium channel in one of two ways. They may cross the cell membrane in the non-ionised form (hence the importance of the concentration of non-ionised drug at the site of action, see below), recharge in the axoplasm and, in this form, enter the ion channel and block it. Alternatively, the non-ionised form may block the ion channel from within the axoplasm itself.

Structural and physicochemical properties

Local anaesthetics have the same basic structure: hydrophilic (usually secondary or tertiary amine) and hydrophobic (usually aromatic) groups separated by an intermediate chain. The classification of local anaesthetic refers to the intermediate chain which can be an ester or an amide. The aromatic and intermediate group may be linked by either an ester or an amide bond. This distinction is important because esters are metabolised rapidly by plasma (and to a lesser extent liver) cholinesterases, and amides more slowly by the hepatic endoplasmic reticulum. Most of the amides, including bupivacaine and ropivacaine but not lignocaine, have a chiral carbon atom, producing R and S steric isomers, and these may differ in their pharmacological properties.

Speed of onset, potency, and duration of action

The speed of onset of local anaesthesia is influenced by the concentration of the non-ionised fraction, the partition coefficient of the free base, and the fraction unbound to protein. The concentration of the non-ionised fraction is determined by the pK_a, the pH of the anaesthetic solution, and the pH at the site of injection. In general, local anaesthetics are weak bases, with pK_a values about 8–9, and are mainly ionised at physiological pH. A low pK_a and high lipid solubility favour a rapid speed of onset. Esters are maintained in a more acidic environment than amides to maintain stability, and so the proportion of drug in the ionised state is higher and the onset relatively delayed. In practice, the speed of onset increases in the order procaine, prilocaine, lignocaine, bupivacaine, and etidocaine.

High lipid solubility is associated with greater potency but *in vivo* other factors may influence apparent potency. For example, lignocaine is twice as potent as prilocaine *in vitro* but there is no difference *in vivo*, probably because lignocaine causes greater vasodilatation and is more rapidly absorbed.

Prolonged duration is associated with high protein binding, slow diffusion from the site of action, and slow vascular uptake.

Pharmacokinetics

In addition to the physicochemical characteristics of the drugs described above, the latency and spread of local anaesthetics are also dependent on dispersion by bulk flow of the injectate and diffusion of the drug to the axon. Volume, speed of injection, dose, baricity, and posture may be important for different sites. Differential onset of block in large myelinated and small unmyelinated nerves is explained partly by delayed diffusion of drug to the axon. In addition, it has been suggested that at least three nodes of Ranvier must be blocked in a myelinated nerve for adequate block, so motor neurons (Aα) with a greater internodal distance are less likely to be blocked than sensory nerves.

Factors important in systemic absorption, and therefore duration, are physicochemistry, vasoactivity, site, dose, addition of vasoconstrictors, and condition of the patient. The more lipid soluble and protein bound drugs such as bupivacaine are associated with slower absorption than, for instance, lignocaine. Increased vascularity at the injection site reduces duration. The addition of adrenaline (usually 1/200 000 or 5 μg/ml) has a greater effect in areas of rapid absorption (e.g. intercostal) and with shorter acting drugs.

Metabolism

The amides are metabolised in the liver by aromatic hydroxylation, *N*-dealkylation, and amide hydrolysis, and the products excreted in the urine. The clearance of prilocaine exceeds liver blood flow indicating a degree of extrahepatic metabolism. Prilocaine is metabolised to *o*-toluidine which may induce methaemoglobinaemia with doses above 600 mg. Hepatic disease may affect significantly the clearance of amide local anaesthetics. The esters are hydrolysed by cholinesterases in the plasma and, to a lesser extent, the liver.

Toxicity

The central nervous and cardiovascular systems are affected primarily. Tinnitus, confusion, vertigo, dysarthria, and palpitations may progress to convulsions, and with higher plasma concentrations, hypotension, respiratory depression and, ultimately, asystolic cardiorespiratory arrest. Blood concentrations associated with significant CNS toxicity are 5–10 μg/ml for lignocaine and 2–4 μg/ml for bupivacaine and etidocaine. The cardiovascular effects are due partly to myocardial depression, caused by reduced sodium entry and therefore decreased calcium release in cardiac muscle, and also vasodilatation, both direct on arterioles and indirect by inhibiting the sympathetic nervous system. Allergic reactions are rare, especially with amides.

Differential motor/sensory block

Bupivacaine exhibits a differential block which is useful in obstetric analgesia and chronic pain. This characteristic reflects a balance between lipid solubility and pK_a, and therefore the ability to block myelinated and unmyelinated fibres. In contrast, etidocaine blocks A- and C-fibres at the same rate, and so motor and sensory block occur together. Ropivacaine demonstrates a significant differential block, which may be useful in obstetric analgesia.

Individual local anaesthetics

Lignocaine

Lignocaine (lidocaine) was the first amino amide to be introduced into clinical practice. It has a rapid onset and duration of about 1–2 hours. Intravenous lignocaine may be useful in neuropathic pain and there are reports of pain relief greatly exceeding the known pharmacological duration of the drug. In this setting the site of action may be either the spinal cord, the DRG, or a peripheral neuroma. Activity in neuromas is inhibited at much lower concentrations than those required for blocking normal peripheral nerve conduction. It is suitable for topical application, and one formulation, EMLA (Eutectic Mixture of Local Anaesthetic), combines 2·5% lignocaine and 2·5% prilocaine. Skin thickness and vascularity are important in determining the speed of onset and duration of analgesia with Emla.

The maximum recommended dose of lignocaine in adults is 200 mg (500 mg with adrenaline).

Prilocaine

Prilocaine is similar in latency and potency to lignocaine, although it causes less vasodilatation and has a longer duration of action. It is the least toxic amide and may be used for intravenous regional anaesthesia. In large doses it may cause methaemoglobinaemia and this precludes its use in obstetrics. The maximum recommended dose for adults is 400 mg. Clinically significant methaemoglobinaemia may occur in adults with doses of >600 mg. It can be treated by intravenous methylene blue 1 mg/kg in a 1% solution.

Bupivacaine

Bupivacaine consists of an optically inactive mixture of its two isomers. It is about four times more potent than lignocaine, and has a longer duration of action (approximately 4–8 hours), although onset is slower. The maximum recommended initial single dose in adults is 150 mg; subsequent doses of 50 mg 2-hourly can be used.

Ropivacaine

Ropivacaine is a new amide which is commercially available as the S isomer. It is similar in its sensory block to bupivacaine at the same dose. Its advantages over bupivacaine are, firstly, greater dissociation between sensory and motor block, which may be important in extradural analgesia during labour, and secondly, lower cardiotoxicity, attributable to the absence of the R isomer.

Antidepressants

Tricyclic antidepressants

The tricyclics are the most widely prescribed group of antidepressants in chronic pain. They were developed in the mid 1950s from a structural modification of the phenothiazine nucleus. The most commonly prescribed tricyclic is amitriptyline, others include imipramine, desipramine, nortriptyline, and doxepin.

Mechanism of action

The tricyclic antidepressants inhibit the reuptake of monoamine neurotransmitters into the presynaptic terminal from the synaptic cleft. The result is facilitation of noradrenergic and serotonergic transmission and the relative effect of individual drugs on these transmitters may vary. For example, desipramine (secondary amine) is a more potent NA reuptake inhibitor than amitriptyline (tertiary amine). On the other hand, amitriptyline has a greater effect on serotonin than desipramine.

Tricyclics have been shown to have beneficial effects in several chronic pain conditions, especially in the management of neuropathic pain. It is believed that these effects are separate to those on mood as pain can be relieved in the absence of depression, with no change in depression rating scales and with relatively low doses. The majority of studies that have demonstrated efficacy of tricyclics in pain control have done so with amitriptyline.

Pharmacokinetics

The tricyclics are rapidly absorbed from the gastrointestinal tract, highly protein bound, and undergo extensive first-pass metabolism in the liver. This involves demethylation, N-oxidation, hydroxylation, and glucuronidation. Active products may be formed, for example amitriptyline is converted to nortriptyline, which has a greater potency for NA reuptake inhibition. Their volume of distribution is very large (approximately 10–50 litres/kg) and half-lives prolonged (amitriptyline $t_{1/2}$ approximately 20 hours). In general, there is wide interindividual variation in steady-state blood concentrations for a given dose.

Pharmacodynamics

These drugs were the first generation of antidepressants and as such have widespread effects on many systems of the body.

Central nervous system

Drowsiness is a common side-effect which the clinician may use to his or her advantage in patients suffering from sleep disturbance. However, even

45

a low dose may cause daytime somnolence as well as dysphoria, agitation, confusion, and aggravation of psychoses.

Autonomic nervous system

Anticholinergic effects are common—dry mouth, constipation, nausea, blurred vision, urinary retention and, rarely, exacerbation of narrow angle glaucoma.

Cardiovascular system

Postural hypotension is more likely in the elderly or patients with cardiovascular disease. Arrhythmias are less common, particularly in low dosage, but reflect their anticholinergic (tachyarrhythmias) or quinidine-like (conduction impairment) properties. They are important in overdose.

Others

Bone marrow depression, skin rashes and photosensitisation, numbness and paraesthesia, fatigue, headache, and hepatic dysfunction have been reported.

Clinical use

Although tricyclics demonstrate a dose–response relation with some types of pain, it is common to start at a low, single daily dose (for amitriptyline, 10 mg over 65 years of age, or 25 mg under 65 years) and increase gradually at 7–10 day intervals. A satisfactory response occurs usually between 25 mg and 75 mg, but occasionally higher. The patient who requires "antidepressant" doses for pain control may, of course, be responding to an improvement in mood, but such a response may also reflect the variable pharmacokinetics of tricyclics between patients. Amitriptyline and doxepin are more sedating, and desipramine and doxepin, less anticholinergic. Lofepramine is less sedative and anticholinergic, and may be safer in overdose.

More selective antidepressants

New types of antidepressants introduced in recent years have had a significant effect on prescribing practice for depression. They include selective serotonin reuptake inhibitors (SSRIs), for example fluoxitine, paroxitine, sertraline, and selective, reversible, monoamine oxidase A inhibitors, for example moclobamide. The SSRIs are structurally different to each other and to the functionally related tricyclic antidepressants. Similarly, moclobamide is structurally different to the monoamine oxidase inhibitors. The new generation are not necessarily more effective than the tricyclics. However, they have fewer side-effects, although the differences are not as great as was once thought. They are generally neither sedating nor stimulating, and have less effect on cholinergic, α-adrenergic, histaminic, and dopaminergic receptors. SSRIs inhibit the cytochrome P-450 system in the liver, which is responsible for the metabolism of tricyclic anti-depressants (TCAs). Therefore, they should be prescribed together with caution.

An important difference between the new and old antidepressants is their half-lives. The new drugs have shorter half-lives than TCAs, particularly moclobamide, and this is important when changing treatment from one antidepessant to another.

Probably, the main advantage with the new antidepressants is that they are much safer in overdose than the TCAs. A fatality following an overdose with the new antidepressants is extremely rare, although they may be lethal in combination with other drugs. There is some evidence that they have analgesic properties, but their efficacy relative to the older antidepressants is not clear.

Anticonvulsants and antiarrhythmics

These drugs stabilise cell membranes by blocking sodium channels and are used primarily in conditions associated with neuropathic pain.

Carbamazepine

Carbamazepine is structurally related to the tricyclic antidepressants. It probably inhibits differentially high frequency neural discharges with no effect on normal conduction. Oral absorption is slow but the bioavailability is 85–100%. It is 75% bound to plasma proteins, and hepatic clearance yields an active metabolite (10, 11-epoxide). Metabolism demonstrates the phenomenon of autoinduction and the initial half-life in the carbamaze-pine-naive subject falls from about 20–50 hours to half that value after a month of treatment. Side-effects are frequent and often limit treatment. They include gastrointestinal upset, headaches, confusion, visual distur-bances, and rash. It has a number of important haematological side-effects including leukopenia, agranulocytosis, and aplastic anaemia, and regular monitoring of blood count is advisable. A low dose, for example 100 mg bd, can be increased slowly until effective, usually 600–800 mg daily. Doses as high as 1600 mg daily may be required in trigeminal neuralgia.

Phenytoin

Phenytoin (diphenylhydantoin) is structurally related to the barbiturates. It has a long unpredictable half-life (7–42 hours) and steady-state plasma concentrations are achieved only after 7–10 days (therapeutic range 10–20 μmol/litre). It is highly protein bound and can be displaced by many drugs, including antidepressants, causing toxicity. It undergoes hydroxylation and conjugation in the liver and the metabolites are excreted in the urine. This enzyme system is saturable and therefore a small increase in dose can lead to a very large increase in plasma concentration. Side-effects include nystagmus, ataxia, slurred speech and other CNS effects, gastro-intestinal and dermatological reactions, osteomalacia, serious haematological disorders, fetal abnormalities and the rare, but potentially fatal, hypersensitivity syndrome.

Dosage should be individualised because of the large interpatient variability. Initially in adults, 3–4 mg/kg/day is recommended, bearing in mind that steady state may not be achieved for 7–10 days.

Sodium valproate

Valproic acid is a derivative of carboxylic acid. It is absorbed rapidly with a high bioavailability. It is 90% protein bound and extensively metabolised in the liver by conjugation and to a lesser extent by oxidation. Some metabolites are potent anticonvulsants. Dosage should start at 600 mg daily and can be increased by 200 mg every 3 days until an effect is achieved. Side-effects are relatively uncommon and usually gastrointestinal but others include rashes, ataxia, tremor, and thrombocytopenia (valproate also inhibits the second stage of platelet aggregation). Fatal liver dysfunction has been reported, particularly in children younger than 3 years on multiple therapy.

Mexiletine

Mexiletine was developed initially as an anticonvulsant. It is a Class Ib antiarrhythmic agent and is structurally similar to lignocaine. It has a high oral bioavailability (85%) with peak plasma concentrations occurring at 2–4 hours. Its elimination half-life is 6–12 hours and it is metabolised in the liver to inactive products. Several prescribing guides have been advocated, including relatively large oral loading doses. However, in the pain clinic a rapid achievement of steady state is probably not necessary and the recommended daily maintenance dose of 600–800 mg in divided doses can be started.

Other drugs

Baclofen

Baclofen (β-(aminomethy)-p-chlorohydrocinnamic acid) is a chemical analogue of the inhibitory neurotransmitter γ-aminobutyric acid (GABA). It depresses monosynaptic and polysynaptic reflex transmission in the spinal cord by activating $GABA_B$ receptors. In neurological diseases associated with painful skeletal muscle spasm, baclofen relieves pain and improves mobility by reducing spasm and clonus.

Baclofen is absorbed rapidly and completely, protein binding is approximately 30%, and half-life 3–4 hours. Its clearance is via the kidneys and only 5% is metabolised.

Baclofen is usually well tolerated, but has a general CNS depressant action. Consequently, side-effects include drowsiness as well as muscle weakness. In addition, headache, visual disturbances, dizziness, seizures, hypotension, bradycardia, nausea, and constipation are observed occasionally.

Baclofen is available for oral and intrathecal administration. A gradual escalating oral dose is recommended and good control of symptoms is often obtained at 20 mg thrice daily.

Intrathecal baclofen may be used when the oral form is ineffective or produces excessive side-effects. A test dose(s) precedes implantation of an intrathecal catheter connected to a suitable implanted infusion pump. Intrathecal doses are about a hundred times less than oral doses and more effective. A mean concentration gradient between lumbar and cisternal CSF of 4:1 occurs at steady-state intrathecal infusion which means that lower limb spasticity can be treated effectively, with little effect on the upper limbs or CNS reactions. Steady state is probably achieved within 1–2 days of a constant rate infusion.

Capsaicin

Capsaicin is the active ingredient of red chilli peppers. It stimulates selectively polynodal nociceptors (C- and thin Aδ-fibres), leading to increased activation of the dorsal horn neurons. Therefore, initial application is algesic. However, repeated application is associated with desensitisation and even blockade of C-fibre conduction. This is the likely explanation for its efficacy in some types of neurogenic pain. The most frequent indication for capsaicin is postherpetic neuralgia, but success has been reported for other conditions in which neuralgic pain is predominant, such as postmastectomy pain and diabetic neuropathy. Improvement may not be observed for 6–8 weeks, and many patients find the burning on skin or even fingers where it is applied to be unacceptable. It is available as a 0·075% cream, to be applied 3–4 times daily.

Selected reading

The following texts offer good reviews of many of the subjects covered in this chapter:

Bonica JJ, ed. *The management of pain*. Philadelphia: Lea and Febiger, 1990.
Fields HL, Lubeskind JL, eds. *Pharmacological approaches to the treatment of chronic pain: new concepts and critical issues*. Seattle: IASP Press, 1995.
Hardman JG, Limbird LE, Molinoff PB, Ruddon RW, Goodman Gilman A, eds. *Goodman*

and Gilman's the pharmacological basis of therapeutics. New York: McGraw-Hill, 1995.

Nimmo WS, Rowbotham DJ, Smith G, eds. *Anaesthesia*. Oxford: Blackwell, 1994.

Wall PD, Melzack R, eds. *Textbook of pain*. London: Churchill Livingstone, 1994.

Wood M, Wood AJJ, eds. *Drugs and anesthesia. Pharmacology for anesthesiologists*. Baltimore: Williams and Wilkins, 1990.

Additional useful papers

Eggars KA, Power I. Tramadol. *Br J Anaesth* 1995;74:247–9.

McClure JH. Ropivacaine. *Br J Anaesth* 1996;76:300–7.

McQuay H, Carroll D, Jadad R, Wiffen P, Moore A. Anticonvulsant drugs for management of pain: a systematic review. *BMJ* 1995;311:1047–52.

Winter J, Bevan S, Campbell EA. Capsaisin and pain mechanisms. *Br J Anaesth* 1995;75:157–68.

3: Postoperative pain and its management

NARINDER RAWAL

Introduction

Despite many advances in our understanding of pain pathophysiology, development of new drugs and sophisticated drug delivery systems, a majority of surgical patients continue to receive inadequate therapy for their postoperative pain. Historically the treatment of postoperative pain has been given low priority by both surgeons and anaesthesiologists. Therefore patients accepted pain as a necessary part of postoperative experience.

Studies conducted since the 1950s have consistently shown that 30–40% of patients report inadequate pain relief or they suffer moderate or severe pain; some studies put the figure as high as 50 or 75%.[1-3] As these studies were largely carried out in centres with a special interest in pain management, it is likely that the problem is even worse in general surgical units. The impression among specialists is that a majority of patients receive unsatisfactory postoperative pain relief.

Barriers to effective postoperative pain relief

The most common method of managing pain after surgery has been and still is the use of intramuscular opioids prescribed on an as needed basis. The inadequacies of this method are well recognized.

Several factors contribute to this problem. Variation in patients' requirements for analgesics may sometimes lead to overmedication but much more commonly to undertreatment. Fluctuating blood levels of analgesic drugs may result in sedation or other adverse effects when the blood levels are high and inadequate analgesia when levels are low before the next injection is given. Another reason for inadequate pain relief by intramuscular opioids is the excessive delay from time of request for pain medication until the nurse is able to respond and administer the prescribed medication. Excessive concerns about side-effects of opioids and about addiction also result in the current undertreatment of postsurgical pain. Other barriers to effective postoperative pain relief are:

- Stoic patient acceptance of pain as an inevitable consequence of surgery in spite of specific questioning revealing that pain may be more severe than anticipated and cause sleep deprivation.
- Lack of quality assurance measures such as frequent pain assessment and its display on bedside chart or nurse station (similar to display of vital signs such as temperature and blood pressure).
- Lack of physician or nurse accountability for inadequate pain treatment.

Furthermore, there is a shortage of clinical teams trained and experienced in the use of new techniques such as PCA and regional analgesia techniques. Some doctors are unfamiliar with specialized PCA administration equipment and are worried about the expense of both the technology and the analgesics it delivers. Epidural technique is highly effective and particularly beneficial in patients undergoing major surgery. However, it requires a high level of technical skill and may be associated with complications such as hypotension, urinary retention, and respiratory depression. Peripheral nerve blocks are safer, simple, and less expensive but are rarely used because of lack of training in the techniques.

Given these problems, it is not surprising that recent surveys from the USA[4] and from a 17-nation European survey[5] revealed that 77% of patients believed that pain was an inevitable postoperative event. Few patients were given information about pain before surgery and a majority experienced severe pain in the first 24 hours after the operation.

Harmful effects of untreated acute pain

Ineffective pain management has significant implications for patient wellbeing. Patients in pain suffer more complications which can lead to a longer hospital stay. There is increasing evidence that improved analgesia may be associated with less morbidity and mortality and with lower costs of hospitalisation.

The pathophysiological consequences of acute pain involve multiple organ systems with alterations in neuroendocrine function, respiration, renal function, gastrointestinal activity, circulation, and autonomic nervous system activity. Untreated severe postoperative pain has several deleterious effects. This is particularly relevant for patients undergoing major thoracic and abdominal surgery. Decreased respiratory movement, splinting, and inability to cough can promote atelectasis and postoperative pulmonary complications. Decreased mobility caused by severe pain makes early ambulation difficult and increases the risk of thromboembolic complications. Severe pain leads to an accelerated catecholamine response and plasma concentrations may be many times normal. The resultant increase in systemic vascular resistance, increased cardiac work and myocardial oxygen consumption may be particularly harmful in patients with coronary arterial disease.

Inadequately treated pain may result in cardiac arrhythmias, hypertension, and myocardial ischaemia. It is well recognised that the risk of myocardial infarction is much higher in the early compared with the late postoperative period. Furthermore, the increased sympathetic activity leads to a significant reduction of blood flow in the lower limbs and an increase in the risk of deep venous thrombosis. Decreases in gastrointestinal motility and in splanchnic circulation may be other detrimental effects of pain-induced catecholamine response.

In the postoperative period pain is widely known to impair coughing and deep breathing leading to small airway closure, intrapulmonary shunting, and hypoxaemia. Postoperative deterioration in pulmonary function appears to be directly related to the proximity of the surgical incision to the diaphragm. Thus patients who undergo upper abdominal or thoracic surgery have considerably more depressed pulmonary function than their counterparts who undergo lower abdominal or extremity surgery. The reduction is less after lower abdominal surgery and is almost negligible following extremity surgery. These pulmonary changes are most pronounced on the first or second day after surgery which is followed by a gradual recovery to preoperative levels in about one week. Since postsurgical pain is believed to be one of the important causes of depressed pulmonary function, effective analgesia can be expected to facilitate earlier return of pulmonary function.

The technique of anaesthesia and postoperative pain management are believed to influence the risk of postoperative thromboembolic complications, especially in patients at high risk such as grossly obese patients and those undergoing hip surgery.[6] Thoracic epidural anaesthesia (TEA) with local anaesthetics has been shown to effectively control severe ischaemic chest pain due to myocardial infarction. The technique has also been used to treat pain in patients with angina pectoris which is resistant to conventional therapy.[7]

Psychological aspects of postoperative pain

All major surgeries confront the patient with the possibility of death. Later this fear is replaced by general anxiety and fear of postoperative pain. Several studies have shown a linear relation between anxiety and postoperative pain. Increasing anxiety and fear lead to increasing pain levels and increased requests for more opioids postoperatively. It has been speculated that these patients treat their anxiety and distress with pain medication.

Although acute pain is often regarded as a single sensation, it is a complex sensation which extends beyond simple nociceptive input. The central processing is modulated by emotive elements such as fear, anxiety, depression, and previous pain experience. The psychological makeup of the patient and the psychological effects of pain should be assessed. Psychological factors that may play a role in exacerbating or diminishing postoperative pain response can be fear and anxiety, sense of loss of control, isolation and fear from normal social supports, learning of cultural and familiar responses to pain, and the individual's prior experience with pain and suffering. There is a great variation in the style of expressing pain. Some patients will not acknowledge pain after major surgery because of high "pain tolerance" or because their coping style does not accept any expression of pain.

There is no direct relation between nociception and pain complaints. The intensity of pain reported by the patient may not accurately reflect underlying nociception. Wide individual responses in pain perception and requirement of analgesics following a particular surgical procedure are commonly seen. It has been reported that 30% of patients undergoing major surgery require no postoperative analgesics. The issue of patient satisfaction is becoming increasingly important as postoperative analgesia delivery systems are left in the hands of the patients. Patient satisfaction regarding postoperative analgesia is a complex issue. Satisfaction ratings are often related more to psychosocial aspects of care such as communication than to technical aspects of care. Patient satisfaction may be directly related to the patients' impression that caregivers are concerned with their analgesia. Studies of patients' satisfaction with pain management reveal that satisfaction with care is seen even when patients report high levels of pain, i.e. satisfaction seems unrelated to the severity of pain.[8] It is generally recognised that patients may have pain but do not tell nurses or doctors. It has been reported that specific questioning of patients who initially reported adequate pain relief revealed that pain had prevented sleep or conversation in these patients.[9]

Pre-emptive analgesia

The concept of pre-emptive analgesia, that pretreatment can prevent pain after surgery or trauma, is based on neurophysiological animal experimental data. There is convincing evidence that acute afferent barrages associated with tissue trauma will generate changes in spinal sensory processing that lead to a hyperalgesic state which may account for the postsurgical pain state. Several clinical studies have evaluated possible pre-emptive analgesic effects by preoperative or intraoperative treatment using regional or local anaesthesia techniques, systemic or epidural opioids, NSAIDs, or paracetamol (acetaminophen).[10] Although some clinical studies have duplicated the impressive results from animal studies, the hypothesis that pretreatment before surgery can significantly reduce postoperative pain and hyperalgesia has generally been a disappointment. Nevertheless, the pre-emptive analgesia debate has focused attention on the importance of using analgesia-based pre- and intraoperative anaesthesia techniques. Surgical stimulation, unlike the experimental models, persists for periods that outlast the effect of treatment. Ongoing nociceptive impulse barrage of the spinal cord neurons from the surgical wound will continue long after the effect of any pretreatment has worn off. It would appear that pre-emptive analgesia will be clinically meaningful only when started before surgery and continued as long as nociceptors are stimulated in the wound area, i.e. several days.[11]

Pharmacology of postoperative pain management

The reader is referred to Chapter 2 for further details.

Broadly, there are three classes of drugs used most commonly to treat postoperative pain. These are opioids, non-opioid analgesics, and local anaesthetic drugs for regional techniques.

Opioid analgesic drugs

Opioids are the most important analgesics in the management of moderate to severe pain. Opioids produce their effect by binding to specific opioid receptors located in the brain, spinal cord, and other areas of the body. Several receptor populations have been identified; for example, mu (μ), kappa (κ), delta (δ), and sigma (σ). It has been proposed that these receptors have their subpopulations, for example that the μ-receptor has two subtypes, μ_1 which mediates analgesia while μ_2 is responsible for respiratory depression and physical dependence. Understandably much research is focused on developing pure μ_1-agonists (Table 3.1). Based on their effects on opioid receptors, opioid drugs may be agonists, antagonists, partial agonists, or agonist-antagonists.

Opioids are still the main drugs for relief of pain. Recent research related to opioids has concentrated on: (i) developing new drugs based on

Table 3.1   Pharmacological profiles of opioid receptors

mu-1 (μ_1)	mu-2 (μ_2)	kappa (κ)	delta (δ)
Analgesia	Analgesia	Analgesia	Analgesia
Supraspinal	—	Supraspinal	Supraspinal
Spinal	Spinal	Spinal	Spinal
—	Respiratory depression	Sedation	Respiratory depression
Euphoria	—	Dysphoria	—
Low addiction potential	Addiction risk	Low addiction potential	Addiction risk
—	Constipation	—	Constipation (minimal risk)
Bradycardia	—	—	—
Hypothermia	—	—	—
Urinary retention	—	Diuresis	—

increased knowledge of opioid receptors and (ii) developing newer drug delivery systems for old drugs based on increasing knowledge of their pharmacokinetics and pharmacodynamics. Many new opioids are more potent but that may not be an advance since a wider margin between analgesia and respiratory depression has been demonstrated.

Several new agonist (alfentanil, sufentanil, remifentanil), antagonist (naltrexone, nalmefene), and agonist-antagonist (nalbuphine, buprenorphine, butorphanol, meptazinol, dezocine) drugs have been introduced recently. The pure agonist opioids alfentanil and sufentanil act on μ-receptors and their analgesic effects are intense and dose related. Both opioids are highly lipophilic, have a short onset of action and fast elimination, and are therefore well suited for administration by infusion. However, these drugs have not been used much by the intravenous route for treating postoperative pain. In contrast, the combination of high receptor affinity and high lipid solubility makes these opioids particularly attactive for epidural administration; both drugs have been used for treating postoperative pain either alone or in combination with local anaesthetic drugs.

Agonist-antagonist opioids

The agonist-antagonist opioids are a heterogeneous group that differs considerably from pure antagonists. These differences are invaluable in understanding opioid action, pain, and addiction. With pure agonists increasing the dose generally causes an increase in analgesia and respiratory depression. Measurement of efficacy is difficult with agonist-antagonist opioids mainly because dose–response relations for these drugs are not linear. In low drug concentration the agonist effect predominates, while in higher concentrations the antagonist effect is predominant. Thus the drug may have low efficacy at higher doses.

Much has been written about the decreased risk of respiratory depression exhibited by these drugs. A "ceiling effect" on respiration has been demonstrated for nalbuphine, buprenorphine, dezocine, and meptazinol. Increasing the dose of opioid will not increase respiratory depression after a certain point—the respiratory depression is believed to reach a plateau. Some of the agonist-antagonist opioids may be safer because of a ceiling effect for respiratory depression but the ceiling also applies to analgesia.[12] In general these drugs have good adverse effect profiles, serious respiratory depression is uncommon, and nausea, constipation, and urinary retention occur less frequently than with morphine. However, serious respiratory depression has been reported after agonist-antagonist drugs.

Of the currently available agonist-antagonists buprenorphine is probably the most widely used. It is a lipophilic agent with high receptor affinity. Its potency is about 25–50 times that of morphine. Its duration of action is about 5–6 hours after intramuscular injection. The drug has excellent absorption by the sublingual route and has been used rather extensively for the management of postoperative and cancer pain. Although a ceiling effect for respiratory depression has been demonstrated in animals, significant respiratory depression may occur with doses used clinically. The non-reversibility of buprenorphine-induced respiratory depression by naloxone has been reported by many. The respiratory stimulant doxapram may be more suitable if respiratory depression occurs after buprenorphine. In summary, although many attempts have been made by the pharmaceutical industry to develop newer analgesic drugs which may possess the analgesic efficacy of morphine but with fewer adverse effects—a "safer morphine"—success has not been achieved so far. At equianalgesic doses the risk of respiratory depression appears to be similar with all agonist opioids. In general none of the current agonist-antagonists represent a major advance on pure agonists. Those with a low risk of respiratory depression also have a low ceiling for analgesia.

Adverse effects of opioids

Table 3.2 shows the possible adverse effects of opioids. With short term, moderate dose opioid treatment as in postoperative pain management, the CNS and gastrointestinal side-effects predominate. Sedation, dizziness, miosis, respiratory depression, nausea, and vomiting appear to be dose dependent. Biliary colic as a result of spasm of the sphincter of Oddi tends to occur more frequently after morphine compared with pethidine administration. Opioids may increase sphincter tone and release anti-diuretic hormone, resulting in urinary retention. Opioid tolerance and physical dependence are unusual in the postoperative setting but can be a problem with chronic opioid treatment. Excessive opioid doses may lead to respiratory depression, apnoea, circulatory collapse, coma, and death. The equianalgesic doses of different opioids are shown in Table 3.3. The two most feared side-effects of opioid administration are respiratory depression and addiction risk.

Opioid addiction, dependence, and tolerance

An important reason for undertreatment of pain is the fear of addiction to opioids. The risk of addiction from therapeutic use of opioids to treat

Table 3.2   Adverse effects of opioids

Organ system	Possible adverse effects
Central nervous system	Sedation, miosis, euphoria, nausea and vomiting, addiction risk
Respiratory system	Respiratory depression, apnoea
Gastrointestinal system	Delayed gastric emptying, constipation
Cardiovascular system	Bradycardia, myocardial depression
Genitourinary system	Urinary retention
Other	Pruritus, allergy

Table 3.3 Analgesic doses of opioids that are equianalgesic with an intramuscular (IM) dose of 10 mg morphine

Opioid	IM dose	Oral dose
Pethidine	100 mg	400 mg
Methadone	8–10 mg	15–20 mg
Morphine	10 mg	30–60 mg
Heroin	3–5 mg	50–60 mg
Codeine	130 mg	200 mg
Hydromorphone	1·5 mg	6–8 mg
Buprenorphine	0·3–0·4 mg	0·4 mg (sublingual)
Nalbuphine	10 mg	—
Butorphanol	2 mg	—

acute pain is extremely rare. Patients receiving opioids during a prolonged period will usually develop *physical dependence*. If the opioid is stopped or greatly reduced in dose the patient may exhibit symptoms of opioid withdrawal. This is different from *psychological dependence* which is associated with drug-seeking behaviour in patients addicted to opioids. *Tolerance* is a decrease in sensitivity to opioids so that escalating doses are required to obtain the same analgesic effect. *Addiction* is chronic and compulsive use of opioids in spite of harmful physical, psychological, and social effects, it is always associated with drug-seeking behaviour.

Non-opioid analgesics

Paracetamol (acetaminophen), aspirin, dipyrone, and non-steroidal anti-inflammatory drugs (NSAIDs) are the most common non-opioid analgesics used to treat mild to moderate postoperative pain as sole agents or in combination with other analgesic drugs such as opioids or techniques such as epidural or peripheral nerve blocks.

Paracetamol (acetaminophen) has an advantage over aspirin in that it does not damage the mucosa of the gastrointestinal tract and does not affect platelet function but it does not provide significant anti-inflammatory activity. The mechanisms of action of paracetamol (acetaminophen) are somewhat controversial; recent evidence suggests that the prostaglandin synthesis is inhibited more centrally rather than peripherally.

NSAIDs

NSAIDs are believed to inhibit COX and synthesis of prostaglandins, thromboxane A_2, and prostacyclin. Prostaglandins that are released due to tissue injury sensitise nerve endings to nociceptive stimuli by lowering the threshold of pain receptors. Recent evidence suggests that NSAIDs also have a central effect in addition to their well-recognised peripheral analgesic actions.[13]

The analgesic efficacy of NSAIDs is quite similar, however, there may be differences in their adverse effect profiles. Although most NSAIDs have been available for oral or rectal administration, they are becoming available also in parenteral form. The latter includes drugs such as indomethacin, diclofenac, suprofen, ketorolac, and tenoxicam. There seems to be a "ceiling effect" to NSAID analgesia, i.e. increasing dosage does not result in improved analgesia. When used with other modalities as part of a "multimodal" analgesic technique, NSAIDs have resulted in 20–60% reduction in opioid requirement. This can be expectd to reduce opioid related morbidity, however, there are no clinical data to support this at present. Non-opioids may be particularly suitable in procedures involving musculoskeletal, post-traumatic, and inflammatory pain in which prostaglandins are known to be pathogenetically involved.

Adverse effects of NSAIDs

In general, adverse effects are infrequent, however, NSAIDs can cause severe complications in the postoperative period. Nausea, dyspepsia, peptic ulceration, perioperative acute renal failure, bleeding disorders, and anaphylactoid reactions have been reported. Advanced age and long term use increase these risks considerably.

Gastrointestinal

Mucosal erosions of the gastrointestinal tract can occur, and this problem is not avoided if NSAIDs are given rectally or parenterally. Gastric irritation and ulceration are less likely if the duration of treatment is only a few days.

Haematological

Reduced platelet aggregation and prolonged bleeding time may occur with aspirin; this effect is "irreversible", i.e. it persists for the life of the platelet (7–10 days). In contrast, inhibition of platelet aggregation by NSAIDs is "reversible", i.e. of shorter duration and lasts only as long as these drugs are in the body.

Renal

Even short term administration of NSAIDs may decrease renal blood flow and glomerular filtration rate resulting in acute renal failure. The risk is higher in patients with known renal disease and extremes of age. Even in otherwise healthy patients the superimposed renal effects of anaesthesia, surgery, hypovolaemia, and dehydration on the risk of NSAID-induced renal failure should be considered.

Other adverse effects

Allergic reactions, bronchospasm, abnormalities in liver function tests, CNS symptoms (headache, dizziness, tinnitus, confusion, drowsiness, depression), and blood dyscrasias have been reported.

Future prospects

Most NSAIDs in current use are inhibitors of both COX-1 and COX-2. Since almost all adverse effects of NSAIDs are due to inhibition of COX-1, development of agents which selectively act on COX-2 will transform the approach to pain management. Selective COX-2 inhibitors are currently under clinical development. Another interesting approach is the peripheral administration of NSAIDs. Promising results have been reported following administration of these drugs in the surgical wound, intra-articularly and in combination with local anaesthetics for peripheral nerve blocks and intravenous regional anaesthesia (IVRA). However, these results need to be confirmed in controlled trials.

Methods of postoperative analgesia

Opioids remain the most useful drugs for treating moderate to severe pain. Table 3.4 shows the methods available to treat postoperative pain.

Table 3.4   Postoperative analgesia techniques

I	**Administration of opioids**
	Intramuscular injection
	Subcutaneous (intermittent bolus injection, continuous infusion)
	Oral (tablets, mixture)
	Patient-controlled analgesia (PCA)
	Rectal
	Intravenous (intermittent bolus, continuous infusion)
	Epidural (intermittent bolus, continuous infusion)
	Sublingual
	Oral transmucosal (Oralet) ("lollipop")
	Transdermal (regular "patch", iontophoresis "patch")
	Intranasal
II	**Administration of non-opioid analgesics**
	Paracetamol (oral, rectal)
	Non-steroidal anti-inflammatory drugs (NSAIDs) (oral, rectal, intramuscular (IM), intravenous (IV), intra-articular)
	Dipyrone (Novalgin) (oral, rectal, IM, IV)
III	**Regional techniques**
	Epidural (local anaesthetics and/or opioids, and/or clonidine)
	Spinal (local anaesthetics and/or opioids, and/or clonidine)
	Paravertebral
	Peripheral nerve blocks
	Wound infiltration
	Interpleural
	Intra-articular (local anaesthetic and/or opioid)
IV	**Non-pharmacological methods**
	Transcutaneous electrical nerve stimulation (TENS)
	Cryoanalgesia
	Acupuncture
V	**Psychological methods**

Opioids can be administered by several routes, each offering advantages and disadvantages (Table 3.5).

Intramuscular administration of analgesics

Postoperative pain has been traditionally managed with intermittent injection of intramuscular opioids. Often a standard dose is prescribed on an "as needed" basis. The standard practice of injecting intramuscular opioids on demand gives poor results due to several reasons. These include

Table 3.5   Advantages and disadvantages of different routes of opioid administration

Method of administration	Advantages	Disadvantages
Oral	Convenient for staff and patients Inexpensive Simple	Absorption slow and variable Impractical after surgery due to risk of vomiting and delayed gastric emptying Problem with first-pass metabolism of morphine
Intramuscular	Convenient for staff Inexpensive	Absorption slow and variable Uncomfortable for patients
Rectal	Feasible when oral or parenteral administration not possible Useful for children	Absorption slow and variable Cultural objections in some countries
Intravenous infusion	Administration simple Guaranteed absorption	Risk of respiratory depression and hypoxia Risk of malfunction with infusion pump Requires careful monitoring
Intravenous bolus (titrated to effect)	Enables individualisation of therapy Inexpensive	Staff training required
Patient-controlled analgesia (PCA)	High patient satisfaction Enables individualisation of therapy	Expensive equipment Risk of malfunction/error Staff training required Strict monitoring (labour intensive)
Epidural opioids	Excellent analgesia at small doses Superior to other methods Improves postoperative outcome in high risk patients	Requires skilled anaesthesiologist Risk of delayed respiratory depression Strict monitoring (labour intensive)
Peripheral nerve blocks	Excellent analgesia Superior to other methods No cardiovascular or respiratory problems	Requires skilled anaesthesiologist

difficulties in quantifying pain, widely varying analgesic requirements depending on type of surgery and location of surgical incision, and on varying pharmacokinetics between individuals. Failure to recognise the extent of pain and fear of precipitating respiratory depression may lead to analgesia being withheld, resulting in irregular administration, fluctuating plasma levels, and hence inadequate pain relief. Intramuscular injections are painful and the technique induces a feeling of dependency on the nursing staff.

Despite these disadvantages, intermittent intramuscular opiates remain the most common method of administering postoperative analgesia. The technique of injecting intramuscular opioids on demand represents familiar practice; generations of nurses have used the technique which may therefore be safe because of accumulated experience. Since no special equipment is required the technique is simple and inexpensive. The gradual onset of analgesia allows observation of the gradual onset of possible overdose. However, too frequently adequate analgesia is not achieved by this approach. Pain is not necessarily constant throughout the postoperative period and an increase in pain may follow movement and physiotherapy. The goal of opioid administration is to find the often narrow therapeutic window between unrelieved pain and excessive sedation and respiratory depression. Drug and dose selection as well as dosing frequency should be individualised. Frequent evaluation of adequacy of pain therapy is important. It should be recognised that properly administered opioids can provide excellent analgesia. With attentive nursing care, appropriate drug and dosing selection, and frequent pain assessment, conventional intramuscular opioid therapy can become "on demand" and may be as effective as PCA (see "Organisation of postoperative pain management services" p 83).

Intravenous analgesic administration

Intravenous infusions

To achieve rapid analgesia in the early postoperative period small boluses of intravenous opioids are commonly administered. Intravenous administration of analgesics delivers a more predictable maximum concentration compared with oral or intramuscular administration, because the absorption process is eliminated. The main advantage is the rapid onset of pain relief. However, intermittent injections will result in wide fluctuations of plasma concentration. Due to rapid decline of plasma levels the analgesic effects may be of short duration and continuous intravenous infusions have been used. Lipophilic opioids with rapid onset of action (fentanyl, alfentanil, pethidine) are preferable to morphine for this route of opioid administration. There is always a risk of respiratory depression, and periods of apnoea associated with arterial desaturation have been reported. The technique should therefore be used only in high-dependency areas. The

Table 3.6   Minimum effective analgesic concentration (MEAC) in plasma for some of the most common opioids

Opioid	MEAC (ng/ml)
Morphine	16
Fentanyl	1
Pethidine	455
Alfentanil	10

technique has been developed further by the additional demand for bolus analgesia and is better known as PCA.

The steady-state plasma concentration of opioids should be kept as close as possible to the minimum effective analgesic concentration (MEAC) in order to achieve effective analgesia. A 4–6-fold interindividual variation may be seen in plasma levels of opioids which provide adequate analgesia. A titrated loading dose followed by maintenance infusion will result in analgesia for as long as the MEAC is exceeded. However, dosage adjustments may be necessary because of interindividual variability in analgesic response. The variability in MEAC may be due to individual differences in production and clearance of endogenous opioids and individual differences in receptor response. The MEAC for some of the most common opioids is shown in Table 3.6. Thus the recommended loading doses for the most common opioids are 5–15 mg for morphine, 50–150 mg for meperidine, and 50–150 mg for fentanyl. The maintenance doses are 1–6 mg/h, 15–60 mg/h, and 30–130 mg/h, respectively. The risk of overdosage should be avoided by careful observations of analgesic response and respiratory function. The infusion equipment should be safe and reliable and personnel should be trained to recognise early signs of inadequate and excessive blood levels.

Intravenously titrated bolus injections

This is an excellent method for obtaining rapid pain relief and is commonly used in postanaesthesia recovery rooms, neonatal units, and burns units. It is also recommended in the management of episodes of "breakthrough pain" or "incident pain" experienced during physiotherapy, dressing changes, and cancer pain therapy. Small doses of opioids are titrated to effect thus achieving the most important goal of pain management, i.e. individualised analgesia. At our institution ward nurses administer 1–2 mg morphine every 4–5 minutes until the pain score is 3 or below on the 10-grade visual analogue scale (VAS). The technique is used when PCA is not indicated or there is a shortage of PCA pumps. The patient is monitored for 30 minutes (bedside nurse presence is not necessary)—a sedation score below 2 (on a 4-grade score) and respiratory rate above 10/min are aimed for. At our institution this technique has replaced intramuscular opioid injection as the most common analgesic technique on all surgical wards. Although pain management by intravenously titrated bolus opioid injections is labour intensive, our nursing staff have accepted this technique because they have experienced that the advantages outweigh the problems due to the somewhat increased workload (see also "Organisation of postoperative pain management services" p 83).

Subcutaneous administration

As with other routes of opioid administration morphine is still the most common opioid for intermittent or continuous subcutaneous administration. Drugs given by this route should be in such concentrations that large volumes are avoided because that may be a cause of local pain. The dosage, uptake of morphine into circulation, clinical effects, and adverse effects are also similar to those following intramuscular morphine administration. A more comfortable alternative for the patient is subcutaneous administration via an indwelling, fine plastic cannula fixed with a transparent dressing below the clavicle or close to the umbilicus. Injections through this indwelling cannula eliminate the need for painful, repeated injections. This technique is commonly used in the treatment of cancer pain, it is also recommended for the management of postoperative pain.

Oral administration

This route is generally regarded as unsuitable for administration of opioids in the early postoperative period because of delay in gastric emptying and consequently lack of absorption of the drug from the small intestine. Oral opioids have a low bioavailability due to first-pass metabolism in the liver. However, these drugs may be useful in treating pain after outpatient surgery and in the late postoperative period when gastrointestinal function has recovered after major surgery.

Slow-release morphine is believed to achieve more sustained blood concentrations than intramuscular morphine and offers the advantage of ease of administration. It is commonly used for the treatment of cancer pain but has no role in postoperative pain because of its slow onset of action. The equianalgesic doses of some of the commonly used analgesics are shown in Table 3.3.

Rectal administration

Treatment of postoperative pain by rectally administered drugs depends greatly on traditions and routines in various countries. Thus it is a common method in Scandinavian countries and France but almost taboo in Greece, Portugal, Ireland, and the UK. The technique is useful in children who dislike the pain and discomfort of intramuscular injection. The absorption of drugs is unaffected by nausea, vomiting, or delay in gastric emptying.

Compared to oral administration this route has the advantage of possible avoidance of the "first-pass" effect since the portal system is bypassed. Morphine and NSAIDs such as diclofenac, ibuprofen, and naproxen have been successfully employed as postoperative analgesics. Morphine in a hydrogel suppository has been used to achieve sustained plasma concentration. Hydrogels are biologically inert and hydrophilic. In the dehydrated form they are firm and can be moulded. When hydrated they swell to two to four times their volume and release drugs in a predictable manner. Oral NSAIDs may cause dyspepsia, gastric erosions, or bleeding; the use of suppositories may reduce these adverse effects. However, the risks are not completely eliminated because gastric irritation is not a local effect only, plasma concentrations of the drug also play an important role. At our institution about 20 000 patients undergo surgery annually and, unless there is a contraindication (liver disease, rectal disease), all patients receive a paracetamol suppository as "base analgesia" every 6 hours. Adults and older children administer the drug themselves. The dosage is 1 g for adults and 15–20 mg/kg for children.

Sublingual administration

Buprenorphine is a potent synthetic agonist-antagonist opioid with a high receptor affinity and slow dissociation constant of drug–receptor complex which permits a prolonged drug effect in the presence of low plasma concentrations. Tablets may be removed from the mouth in the event of overdosage, also accidental swallowing does not result in toxicity because of the high first-pass hepatic metabolism and resultant low bioavailability. The major disadvantages are a relatively high degree of sedation and nausea; respiratory depression when it occurs can be severe and prolonged and is not reversible by naloxone.

Oral transmucosal route

Fentanyl incorporated into a candy matrix and formulated in a lollipop is a novel method of opioid administration. Studies in adult volunteers have shown that oral transmucosal fentanyl produces dose-dependent increases in sedation and analgesia. These fentanyl lollipops have also been used successfully for premedication in children. Doses around 15–20 mg/kg appear satisfactory. However, the incidence of adverse effects such as facial pruritus and nausea was high. Larger doses were associated with considerable respiratory depression and an extemely high incidence of pruritus, nausea, and vomiting. The concept of administering opioids via a non-threatening and psychologically appealing delivery system appears attractive. Current data suggest that the palatable lollipops are readily accepted by children. In the USA, fentanyl lollipops are marketed under the name Oralet. Further studies are necessary to confirm if this novel method has a wider application for premedication and postoperative analgesia.

Intranasal administration

The nasal route is less traumatic than intramuscular injection, is more aesthetic than rectal administration, and may be particularly acceptable to children. Butorphanol, fentanyl, and sufentanil have been administered intranasally to treat moderate to severe pain. Both drugs have also been used for premedication. Intranasal cocaine has been known to drug addicts for a long time. In recent years other drugs such as midazolam, ketamine, and nitroglycerine have been used in anaesthesiology. Sufentanil is preferred to fentanyl because smaller volumes are required due to the higher potency of the drug. Sufentanil in a total dose of 10–20 µg and doses of 1·5–3 µg/kg has been shown to provide effective preoperative sedation of rapid onset. However, in children receiving larger doses (4·5 µg/kg) intranasal sufentanil was associated with vomiting, a marked decrease in ventilatory compliance, muscular rigidity, and convulsive activity. At our institution, fentanyl 1 µg/kg is frequently used to treat pain in the recovery room in situations where the child has pulled out the intravenous line. Intranasal fentanyl is not associated with the burning sensation that is reported with other drugs such as sufentanil and midazolam.

Patient-controlled analgesia (PCA)

Along with intraspinal opioids, PCA represents the most significant recent advance in the management of pain. PCA with intermittent intravenous doses of opioids was first described by Sechzer in 1968.[14] It is a technique that allows patients to treat their pain by directly activating doses of analgesics. The patient controls the rate of drug administration (within prescribed limits) to achieve immediate pain relief. The concept of PCA permits the patients to correct for individual differences in tolerance, variability in pharmacokinetics, or inappropriate "screening" by nursing or medical staff. PCA allows patients to maintain adequate analgesia regardless of changes in pain intensity over time. It has been demonstrated by many workers that patients self-administer analgesic medications appropriately and responsibly, that they titrate opioids effectively, and, in fact, that the total analgesic dose requirements are less than those with intramuscular opioid. PCA has achieved widespread acceptance as an analgesic modality for improving postoperative and labour pain as well as chronic pain and cancer pain. It can also be used as a research tool to determine equipotency ratio between analgesics and between routes of administration of different analgesics.

Although the concept of PCA theory was introduced nearly 30 years ago, recent progress in the apparatus and microprocessor technology has renewed interest in this modality. Unlike other modes of opioid administration, with PCA the patient determines the dose required to maintain adequate analgesia. The optimum plasma concentration is that which satisfies the patient's subjective requirement of pain relief while avoiding excessive drug which may be associated with adverse effects.

Although the MEACs of various opioids are known (Table 3.6), there is a considerable interindividual variation in the plasma concentration time profile between patients. Several pharmacokinetic factors may be responsible for variability in response to drugs, these include drug dose, age, gender, body weight, disease states (renal, hepatic, cardiac), and genetic polymorphism. The titrating of drug dose to clinical effect is therefore extremely important.

PCA modes and dosing parameters

There are several PCA systems on the market and include devices manufactured by Abbott, Bard, Baxter, Braun, Graseby, Ivac, and Pharmacia. These systems incorporate a microprocessor that allows the patient to interact with an infusion pump connected to the intravenous line.

Demand dosing Patients activate the pump by pressing a button connected to the apparatus. A pre-programmed fixed amount of analgesic drug is then administered over 10–30 seconds. A *lock-out interval* is begun after each injection; this prevents a second dose being delivered within a preset time interval. Depending on the drug and dosage selected the lock-out interval usually is in the range of 5–15 minutes (Table 3.7).

Constant-rate infusion plus demand dosing Here the minimum or background administration rate is prescribed by the physician; however, this mode allows the patient to supplement the dose.

Variable-rate infusion plus demand dosing A microprocessor monitors

Table 3.7 Demand dose and lock-out intervals for PCA with some of the commonly used opioids

Opioid	Concentration	Demand dose	Lock-out interval (min)
Morphine	1 mg/ml	0·5–3 mg	5–12
Fentanyl	10 μg/ml	10–20 μg	5–10
Pethidine	10 mg/ml	5–30 mg	5–12
Methadone	1 mg/ml	0·5–2·5 mg	8–20
Hydromorphone	0·2 mg/ml	0·05–0·25 mg	5–10
Nalbuphine	1 mg/ml	1–5 mg	5–10

demand and controls the infusion rate accordingly.

Loading dose This is the physician-administered dose prior to initiation of PCA. To achieve optimal MEAC in plasma (Table 3.6), the natural accumulation time of four half-lives can be bypassed by administration of a loading dose. This is usually a relatively large bolus given in divided intravenous doses and titrated to effect. This loading dose enables plasma concentrations to reach a level where maintenance PCA doses can sustain a steady state.

The Baxter PCA Infusor is a simple and small non-electronic device which is disposable. The device is non-programmable, it delivers a fixed dose at fixed intervals via a balloon reservoir that deflates slowly. The Abbott, Bard, Baxter, and Pharmacia devices are all suitable for ambulatory use. The on-demand technique has also been used for other routes of opioid administration such as oral PCA, intramuscular PCA, sublingual PCA, subcutaneous PCA, and epidural PCA.

With increasing experience it is becoming clear that PCA provides a better quality of analgesia than that provided by conventional intramuscular or intravenous opioids. The choice of drug appears to be of lesser importance. The choice of opioid may depend on local traditions, some opioids are used almost exclusively in certain countries, for example diamorphine in the UK and Ireland, ketobemidone in Scandinavian countries, piritramide in Germany and Austria, nicomorphine in the Netherlands and Belgium, oxycodone in Finland. Table 3.8 shows the choice of opioids in a 17-nation European survey.[15] Given the marked pharmacodynamic variability in the analgesic requirements of patients, the bolus dose and lock-out interval may have to be altered occasionally to optimise therapy. To achieve optimal results both the patient and the nursing staff should understand the basic principles upon which the technique is based. Patients should be instructed on the use of the PCA device prior to the initiation of therapy. The concept of PCA has also been applied to the management of labour pain, acute pain of myocardial infarction, and in clinical research. An important psychological advantage of PCA is its ability to reduce the delay between the perception of pain and the administration of analgesic medication. The on-demand technique has also been used for other routes of opioid administration such as intramuscular PCA, sublingual PCA, subcutaneous PCA, and epidural PCA. PCA is a useful research instrument for the study of analgesics and analgesia techniques because the method provides the researcher with an objective index of analgesic need.

PCA is widely used in the USA. Even in Europe its use has increased considerably in recent years. The 17-nation European survey showed that PCA was routinely used to treat postoperative pain in 67% of the 105 hospitals surveyed.[15] Of the 836 000 inpatients undergoing surgery during

Table 3.8   Choice of opioids for PCA in Europe: data from a 17-nation survey of 105 hospitals. (Reproduced with permission from Rawal N. Patient-controlled analgesia (PCA) for postoperative pain—a European survey. *Reg Anesth* 1995;74:134)

Austria	M > Pir
Belgium	M, Pir > F
Denmark	M
Finland	O > M, F
France	M
Germany	Pir
Greece	—
Iceland	—
Ireland	M
Italy	M > B
The Netherlands	M > N
Norway	M
Portugal	M
Spain	M
Sweden	M
Switzerland	M > T
UK	M > D
Mean	M > Pir > O > F > B, D, N, T

M = morphine; Pir = piritramide; F = fentanyl; O = oxycodone; B = buprenorphine; N = nicomorphine; T = tramadol; D = diamorphine.

one year, 11% (89 000 patients) received PCA. It has a high degree of patient acceptance. There is no evidence that there is increased risk of adverse effects. This is partly because overmedication with opioids usually leads to sedation which typically precedes respiratory depression. A sedated patient cannot self-administer additional opioid. However, cases of severe respiratory depression due to operator or equipment error have been reported. It must be realised that although PCA pumps in general have an excellent safety record, they are mechanical devices and may break down. In the 17-nation European survey, 17 cases of respiratory depression (0·02%) were noted.[15] Of these, five cases were due to malfunction of equipment leading to overdosage. Malfunction of a PCA device causing massive overdose resulting in respiratory arrest and death has been reported. There are anecdotal reports of respiratory depression following activation of PCA devices by patients' visitors. This unauthorized activation bypasses the inherent safety feature of PCA by which, as patients become more sedated, they are unable to press the button and therefore cannot give themselves a bolus dose. Supervision by trained nursing personnel is therefore extremely important. Preoperativae teaching of PCA must also emphasise that the patient is the only person who should activate the pump. PCA should be used cautiously in elderly and high risk patients and in patients with hypovolaemia. In small children and in patients with psychiatric disease, appropriate self-dosing may be difficult.

The rationale for a continuous infusion of opioid is that the patient requires fewer bolus doses allowing patients to sleep for longer periods and reducing or eliminating painful episodes that wake up the patient. However, current evidence about these beneficial effects of continuous infusion is inconclusive. This technique does not always result in improved analgesia or better sleep. It does not take into consideration the fact that postoperative pain intensity decreases with time. Since it is not truly "patient controlled" it reduces the inherent safety of PCA because the opioid is delivered whether the patient needs it or not. An increased risk of adverse effects, especially respiratory depression due to excessive doses and questionable advantages, has led many to abandon the use of continuous background infusion mode for PCA. However, this technique may be beneficial in patients requiring PCA for long periods and for cancer pain.

Monitoring routines for PCA vary considerably. In general, respiratory rate and sedation level should be monitored at regular intervals in all patients receiving opioids for acute pain. At our institution this is done every hour (the same monitoring as for epidural opioids). However, in several institutions less strict monitoring is practised. It is relatively common to monitor every 1–2 hours for the first 8–12 hours and then increase the observation interval to 2–4 hours. More frequent and closer observation is required for risk patients such as patients with compromised pulmonary or cardiac function, grossly obese patients, and those with sleep apnoea. Increasingly, pulse oximetry is being used in addition to the above parameters.

Patient-controlled epidural analgesia (PCEA)

The increasing popularity of the intravenous PCA technique in pain management has generated interest in the use of epidural opioids via a PCA pump. This technique allows the patient to self-titrate epidural opioid or an opioid–local anaesthetic combination to the desired level of analgesia. Epidural PCA can be expected to combine the flexibility and convenience of PCA with the superior analgesia of epidural opioids. PCEA can be used as an investigational tool to eliminate bias regarding opioid administration. It has also been suggested that PCEA with opioids results in a more rapid recovery and shorter hospitalisation than intravenous PCA or intramuscular opioids. Because of high lipophilicity and consequent rapid onset, drugs such as fentanyl, sufentanil, and alfentanil have been studied for epidural PCA. A bolus of 10–30 µg sufentanil followed by a basal infusion rate of 5 µg/h with a 5 µg demand dose and a 10–20 minute lock-out interval have been recommended.

Transdermal PCA

Currently available PCA devices are expensive and require ongoing maintenance. Some devices are bulky, which may delay early ambulation.

Many are perceived as complex to programme, increasing the risk of dose error. There is a great potential for developing PCA techniques which are more flexible and easier to use. One such approach under investigation is the transdermal administration of opioids by electrotransport. Pressing a button on a skin patch starts active transdermal transport of the opioid by iontophoresis. Transfer of ionised drugs can be facilitated by a small current across two electrodes: one above the drug reservoir and the other at a distal skin site. The dose can be adjusted by the delivery current; to avoid a depot effect, drug delivery can be stopped by switching off the current. Preliminary results with fentanyl and morphine are encouraging; the product is expected on the market soon. By offering an important alternative to traditional approaches to PCA this modality has the potential to make the PCA technique more widely available.

Regional techniques for postoperative analgesia

The use of parenteral opioids for treating postoperative pain is associated with several adverse effects such as sedation, respiratory depression, nausea, and depression of gastrointestinal function. By avoiding opioids regional anaesthetic techniques provide excellent analgesia in an alert, cooperative patient untroubled by nausea.

Regional anaesthesia techniques are among the most effective and versatile means of providing relief of acute pain. Single injection techniques may be useful after outpatient and minor surgery. In the hospitalised patient who has undergone a more extensive surgical procedure, a catheter (continuous) technique is preferable.

Epidural analgesia

Of all the techniques available for postoperative pain relief none provides greater versatility than epidural block with catheter technique. Analgesia can be provided from upper chest to toes. Epidural block is increasingly a part of the anaesthetic technique; the catheter can be used to extend the block during the postoperative period. Local anaesthetics or opioids or a combination of these drugs will provide excellent postoperative analgesia.

In the literature there is convincing evidence regarding the role of epidural block in improving pulmonary function, increasing lower limb blood flow, reducing the incidence of thromboembolic complications, attenuating neuroendocrine stress response to surgery, decreasing myocardial oxygen demand, and stimulating intestinal motility. Patients who have undergone major thoracic or abdominal surgery are prone to pulmonary complications because pain prevents them from breathing deeply and coughing effectively. The abolition of pain by epidural block might be expected to improve pulmonary function. However, the effects of epidural analgesia are not as dramatic as might be expected. Some improvement in

71

FRC and vital capacity (VC) may be seen but the results are not consistent and improvement is limited to reduction of deterioration rather than restoration of preoperative values.

Despite the above-mentioned advantages the technique has not been widely practised, mainly because the epidural catheter must be placed in the mid-thoracic region for reliable analgesia after thoracic and upper abdominal surgery. This is considerably more exacting than lumbar placement. Close surveillance of the patient is necessary because of the risk of hypotension after every top-up with local anaesthetic. The use of continuous infusion technique with low dose local anaesthetics or with opioids or with combinations of very low doses of both to exploit the synergistic effects of both groups of drugs, has created renewed interest in epidural analgesia for management of postoperative pain. For some patients, the additional analgesia with epidural opioids may be of critical importance. This is particularly true when severe pain may compromise pulmonary function leading to atelectasis and pneumonia. Examples include patients with rib fractures or pain resulting from abdominal or thoracic incisions. Those with underlying medical conditions such as respiratory insufficiency or obesity may also derive particular benefit from best available analgesia. In such situations the need for profound analgesia is of major importance and may make epidural opioids the preferred choice.

Contraindications

The two main contraindications to placement of needles or catheters in the epidural space are:

1 Local or generalised sepsis due to the rare but serious risk of infection of the epidural space, and epidural abscess.
2 Coagulation disorders or anticoagulant therapy due to the equally serious risk of epidural haematoma.

A relative contraindication is hypovolaemia if local anaesthetic drugs are administered, since the sympathetic block by these drugs (as opposed to opioids) can be expected to increase the risk of hypotension.

Choice of drugs for epidural analgesia

The two main categories of drugs used in clinical practice are local anaesthetics and opioids (Table 3.9). In recent years a third category, i.e. α_2-agonists such as clonidine, has also become popular in some institutions.[16]

Epidural local anaesthetic drugs

These drugs are used to provide anaesthesia during surgery and (in low concentrations) analgesia during the postoperative period and for labour

Table 3.9 Differences between local anaesthetic and opioid epidural analgesia

	Epidural local anaesthetic	Epidural opioid
Motor block	Yes	No
Sensory block	Yes	No
Sympathetic block	Yes	No
Adverse effects		
Hypotension	Yes	No
Respiratory depression	No	Yes (early and delayed)
Pruritus	No	Yes
Urinary retention	Yes	Yes
Gastrointestinal motility	Increased	Decreased
Sedation	No	Yes/no*

* Yes = lipophilic opioids; no = morphine.

pain. Epidural administration of these drugs will lead to a sensory, motor, and sympathetic blockade; the intensity of this blockade will depend on the concentration and total dose of the local anaesthetic used. The siting of the epidural catheter in the dermatomal segment that covers the surgical area, i.e. thoracic epidural for chest surgery, is crucial. In general low concentrations of local anaesthetic drugs are used for postoperative analgesia.

Sympathetic blockade may lead to hypotension; its severity depends on the dose of local anaesthetic and the number of segments blocked. Although some degree of hypotension is almost invariably associated with epidural block, significant hypotension is unlikely with the low concentrations ($\geqslant 0.1\%$ bupivacaine) commonly used. However, even in the normovolaemic patient there is some risk of postural or orthostatic hypotension.

Numbness and motor weakness due to sensory and motor block are the other major side-effects of epidural technique with local anaesthetics. Since these are also dependent on concentration and total dose it is not surprising that low concentrations of local anaesthetic drugs are routinely used in the postoperative period. It has been shown that combinations of epidurally administered local anaesthetic drugs and opioids have additive or synergistic analgesic effects. There is some evidence that a combination of low concentration of local anaesthetic and an opioid reduces the adverse effects of each class of drug while providing better analgesia at rest and, more importantly, during mobilisation, coughing, etc. At our hospital such combination therapy consisting of 0.0625% (0.625 mg/ml) bupivacaine and 1 mg/ml sufentanil given at the rate of 5–8 ml/h and with the possibility of a patient activated bolus administration (epidural PCA) has been routinely used since 1993 for labour analgesia. The concentration of local anaesthetic is so low that it allows the parturient to stand and walk, with assistance.

73

Ropivacaine is a new local anaesthetic with a similar pharmacokinetic profile to that of bupivacaine. In contrast to peripheral nerve block, epidural use of ropivacaine provides less intense motor block which is of shorter duration than that following equal concentration of bupivacaine. If injected intravenously ropivacaine is less likely to produce CNS and cardiovascular adverse effects than bupivacaine, suggesting that ropivacaine can be used with greater safety at higher doses. Preclinical data indicate that ropivacaine has a dose-dependent separation of sensory and motor block at low concentration. This can provide effective epidural analgesia with minimal and non-progressive motor block, which may be particularly useful for pain relief during labour and after surgery.

Epidural opioid drugs

The discovery of opioid receptors has opened new horizons in pain management. By bypassing the blood and the blood–brain barrier, small doses of opioids administered in either the subarachnoid or epidural spaces provide profound and prolonged segmental analgesia. This undoubtedly represents a major breakthrough in pain management. Since their introduction into clinical practice in 1979,[17, 18] spinal opioids have achieved great international popularity in a variety of clinical settings either as sole analgesic agents or in combination with low dose local anaesthetic. Numerous studies have shown that spinal opioids can provide profound postoperative analgesia with less central and systemic adverse effects than opioids administered systematically. Segmental analgesia induced by intraspinal opioids has a role in the management of a wide variety of surgical and non-surgical painful conditions. The technique has been employed successfully to treat intraoperative, postoperative, traumatic, obstetric, chronic, and cancer pain.

The unique feature of spinal opioid analgesia is the lack of sensory, sympathetic, or motor block, which allows patients to ambulate without the risk of orthostatic hypotension or motor incoordination usually associated with local anaesthetics administered epidurally or opioids administered parenterally. These advantages of spinal opioids are particularly beneficial in high risk patients undergoing major surgery, patients with compromised pulmonary or cardiovascular function, grossly obese patients, and elderly patients.

When an opioid is administered in the epidural space it has to cross the dura before reaching the opioid receptors in the spinal cord. In addition to the physical barrier presented by the dura, the epidural space is highly vascularised and also contains a variable amount of fat and connective tissue. These factors influence the pharmacokinetics of epidurally administered opioids. Depending on the lipophilicity of the opioid, a certain portion of the drug enters the CSF and spinal cord after crossing the dura, a certain portion enters the systemic circulation via epidural veins and a

Table 3.10   Lipid solubility, doses, onset, and analgesia duration of the most common opioids for epidural administration (data are from different studies and therefore not strictly comparable)

Opioid	Lipid solubility*	Bolus dose†	Onset (min)	Duration (h)
Morphine	1	2–5 mg	30–60	12–24
Hydromorphone	1·4	1·0–1·5 mg	20–30	6–12
Diamorphine	10·0	2–6 mg	10–15	6–12
Pethidine	28·0	25–75 mg	10–20	4–8
Methadone	82·0	6–8 mg	10–20	4–8
Fentanyl	580	50–100 μg	10–15	2–4
Sufentanil	1270	20–50 μg	5–10	2–4

* Octanol partition coefficient in relation to morphine.
† Doses should be reduced for elderly and high risk patients.

certain portion binds to epidural fat. Lipophilicity facilitates systemic absorption of opioids.

In general highly lipid soluble drugs such as fentanyl and sufentanil have a more rapid onset and shorter duration of effect than hydrophilic drugs such as morphine (Table 3.10). The hydrophilic opioids are cleared slowly from CSF, resulting in high concentrations of the drug spreading rostrally with the bulk flow of CSF and saturating the entire length of the spinal cord. Thus, administration of epidural morphine at the caudal or lower lumbar level will provide analgesia for upper abdominal or thoracic surgery. In contrast, lipophilic opioids such as fentanyl and sufentanil provide a more segmental analgesic effect, therefore the efficacy of these opioids is dependent on the siting of the epidural catheter.

The long duration of analgesia of epidural morphine allows it to be used as an intermittent bolus twice a day, whereas opioids such as fentanyl and sufentanil are better suited for continuous infusion because of their short duration of analgesia.

Adverse effects of epidural opioids

Some of the reported adverse effects of epidural opioids such as nausea, vomiting, somnolence, and early respiratory depression are dose dependent and are believed to be due to the vascular uptake into systemic circulation. The characteristic adverse effects of epidural opioids are pruritus, urinary retention, and late onset respiratory depression.

Pruritus   The reported incidence of itching following opioids is quite variable, the probable reason is that if not asked specifically the majority of patients do not complain about this complication because of its mild nature. The risk of severe, distressing itching is extremely low. Pregnant patients appear more at risk irrespective of the opioid administered. Patients treated for malignant or chronic pain with epidural or intrathecal opioids do not experience pruritus after the first or second day, presumably because of rapid development of tolerance.

The exact mechanism for epidural opioid-induced pruritus is unclear; it is presumed to be centrally mediated due to activation of μ-receptors. Small doses of naloxone can be used to treat pruritus without reversing analgesia. Other opioid antagonists such as naltrexone and nalmefene, antihistaminic drugs, agonist-antagonist opioids such as butorphanol and nalpuphine, and subhypnotic doses of the anaesthetic induction agent propofol have all been successfully used to treat pruritus.

Urinary retention It is difficult to establish the incidence of urinary retention since a majority of patients who receive epidural analgesia are patients undergoing major surgery who are usually catheterised. Cystometric studies have demonstrated that irrespective of dose epidural morphine reduces the strength of detrusor contraction leading to a corresponding increase in bladder volume. These changes can be prevented and reversed by naloxone. However, if naloxone is given in large doses the reversal of urodynamic effects of epidural morphine will be achieved at the cost of partial or complete reversal of analgesia. In general, if patients are unable to void 6 hours after surgery a single in-and-out catheterisation is indicated to prevent myogenic bladder damage because of prolonged overdistention.

Respiratory depression One of the major advantages of epidural versus parenteral opioid administration is the greatly reduced risk of respiratory depression. Indeed, the most common indication for epidural opioids is the management of postoperative pain in high risk patients undergoing major surgery. However, delayed respiratory depression occurring several hours after opioid administration is the most serious side-effect of this technique. Delayed respiratory depression is believed to result from rostral spread of opioids in the CSF to the brain stem and respiratory centre.

Today we have better understanding of the pattern of respiratory depression. It is slow and progressive in onset rather than a sudden apnoeic event. It should be noted that respiratory rate alone is unreliable for establishing the presence or lack of respiratory depression. Monitoring of level of consciousness (usually on a 4-grade scale) is important since increasing sedation is associated with advancing respiratory depression. The belief that lipophilic opioids (fentanyl, sufentanil, pethidine) are safer than morphine because they do not spread rostrally in the CSF is being increasingly questioned. Delayed respiratory depression after epidural opioids is extremely rare (0.1–1%), unpredictable, and can occur with any opioid. As with opioids administered by any route the risk of respiratory depression after epidural opioids is increased with large doses of opioids, advanced age, concomitant use of systemic opioids and/or sedatives, high

Table 3.11   Risk factors for respiratory depression following epidural or intrathecal opioid administration

---

Large doses (>5 mg epidural morphine, >0·3–0·4 mg intrathecal morphine)
Advanced age
High risk patients (according to ASA classification)
Opioid naive patients
Concomitant administration of other analgesics or sedatives
Thoracic opioid administration (vs lumbar)?

---

risk patients, and opioid naive patients (Table 3.11). It is generally accepted that all patients receiving epidural opioids should be monitored for at least 12 hours after epidural morphine, less after lipophilic opioids. If trained staff can monitor respiratory rate and sedation frequently (every hour), there is no reason why the patients cannot be nursed on regular surgical wards.

Epidural non-opioid drugs

Non-opioid receptor selective agents such as serotoninergic, muscarinic, adenosinergic, GABA, somatostatin agonists, and SP antagonists are believed to inhibit pain modulation at the spinal level. In clinical practice analgesic effects have been demonstrated following epidural or intrathecal administration of non-opioids such as clonidine, somatostatin, octreotide, ketamine, calcitonin, midazolam, droperidol, and neostigmine. However, with the exception of the α_2-agonist clonidine these drugs are largely experimental at present. A synergism between α-adrenergic and opioid systems has been proposed. Epidural clonidine has been shown to reduce opioid requirements in postoperative patients, it also prolongs the duration of analgesia achieved by epidural opioids such as morphine, fentanyl, or sufentanil.

Combination of local anaesthetics and opioids

The rationale for the combination technique is that these two types of drugs eliminate pain by acting at two distinct sites, the local anaesthetic at the nerve axon and the opioid at the receptor site in the spinal cord. Spinal opioids alone provide good pain relief at rest but may not be adequate during physiotherapy and mobilisation. Patients receiving a combination of a low dose local anaesthetic and opioid have a more rapid onset of analgesia, more profound and longer-lasting pain relief, and less motor blockade than patients receiving either drug alone. For example, patients undergoing knee replacement surgery are not immediately ambulatory in the early postoperative period; these patients are uniquely suited for an analgesic regimen that includes some degree of neural blockade that facilitates vigorous physical therapy and continuous passive motion of the

JET LIBRARY

operated knee. Combination therapy as continuous infusion or as epidural PCA ("walking epidural") (Fig. 3.1) has been extensively studied in the obstetric population. The practice of adding local anaesthetic to opioid has been questioned by some. In some studies the combination did not improve analgesia and in fact was associated with increased morbidity. Local anaesthetics have the potential to cause side-effects such as hypotension, motor weakness, urinary retention, and pressure sores due to skin sensory loss. The optimum combination that has opioid-sparing synergistic effect without delaying mobilisation is yet to be established.

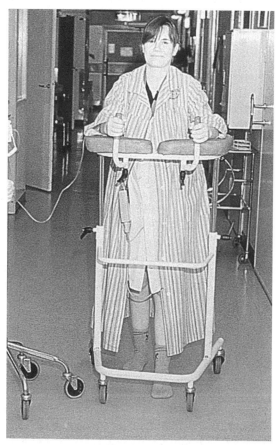

Fig 3.1 The use of a "walking epidural" for labour pain. The use of combination of low doses of local anaesthetics and opioids is being increasingly used to provide epidural analgesia for labour, postoperative, and cancer pain. The dose of local anaesthetic can be reduced to such an extent that it is possible for patients to ambulate (with assistance)—so called "walking epidural". (Reproduced with permission from Rawal N. *Smärtlindring med epidurala och intratekala opioider.* Trycksak nr PPS 660, 1996;43)

Other regional techniques for postoperative analgesia

Wound infiltration

Wound infiltration is perhaps the simplest method for providing wound analgesia but is all too frequently neglected. Perfusion of local anaesthetic through an indwelling catheter under the rectus sheath to treat post-laparotomy pain was described almost 40 years ago.

Infiltration of long-acting local anaesthetic into the edges of surgical wounds and implantation of polyethylene catheters in the surgical wound, followed by infusion of local anaesthetics, have been shown to provide effective analgesia. Fears have been expressed that injections of local anaesthetics into the wound may interfere with normal reparative processes. However, there is no evidence to support the concern that wound healing is delayed or infection is introduced by this technique. Topical anaesthetics applied to mucosal surfaces after tonsillectomy provide effective post-operative pain relief.

Plain bupivacaine 0·25% is the preferred local anaesthetic. Adrenaline-containing local anaesthetics should be avoided due to the theoretical risk of delayed wound healing. Although the technique has been studied mainly in patients undergoing minor orthopaedic and plastic surgery, it may have a morphine-sparing effect in the control of pain following major surgery. The technique is so simple and effective that it is always worth reminding the surgeon towards the end of surgery that considerable analgesia can be provided by the administration of local anaesthetic into the wound edges.

Recently, a technique has been described which allows day surgery patients to self-administer local anaesthetics in the home environment. Depending on the surgical procedure, catheters are placed in the surgical wound, axillary brachial plexus sheath (hand surgery), subacromially (shoulder surgery), or close to the peritoneum (iliac crest bone graft, maxillofacial surgery); these catheters are connected to a disposable, elastometric (balloon) pump. By opening and closing a clamp on the tubing the patient self-administers a prescribed dose of local anaesthetic when necessary.[19] The technique is undergoing controlled trials.

Peripheral nerve blocks

Any peripheral nerve block (brachial plexus, sciatic, femoral) performed with a long-acting local anaesthetic such as bupivacaine provides analgesia which may last about 12 hours. Wrist, ankle, and elbow blocks are easy to perform. Equally simple and effective are ilioinguinal and iliohypogastric blocks following herniorraphy and intercostal block following upper abdominal or thoracic surgery. In general, appropriate blocks exist for almost all areas of the body (Fig 3.2). Catheter techniques have been described for several peripheral blocks. Catheters can be introduced into the brachial plexus, femoral nerve lumbar pluxus, and intercostal space.

Intercostal block

This is a simple and effective block which has been extensively used to provide pain relief after upper abdominal and thoracic surgery. Overwhelming evidence indicates that the block reduces the requirements of opioids and improves postoperative pulmonary function. The reported duration of analgesia after a single block with 0·5% bupivacaine varies from 3 to 18 hours. Intercostal block is believed to be superior to thoracic epidural block, because it is easier to perform and is not associated with the well-known problems of epidural block such as hypotension, motor weakness, or urinary retention. The major disadvantage of the technique is the need for repeating the block and the risk of pneumothorax. However, the risk of this complication is very low.

Continuous intercostal anaesthesia via an indwelling catheter has been used successfully to treat pain following upper abdominal surgery and chest trauma. The obvious advantage is provision of prolonged analgesia without

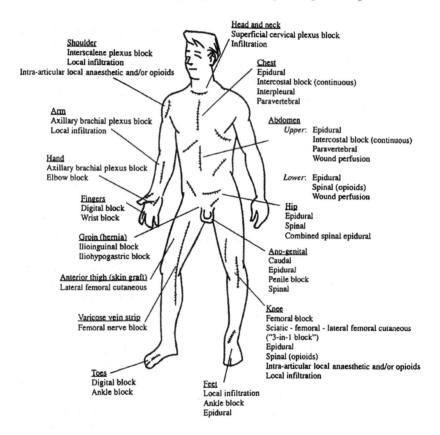

Fig 3.2   Possible regional techniques for the management of postoperative pain

the need for multiple blocks and their attendant risks. Administration of local anaesthetic through a catheter in the intercostal space will block several segments. The technique is also useful for treating pain associated with fractured ribs.

Caudal block

Caudal anaesthesia is probably the most common regional anaesthetic technique for surgery below the umbilicus and for postoperative analgesia in children. It is generally considered to be a simple, safe, and effective block. (See Chapter 5 for details about caudal and other regional blocks.)

Transcutaneous electrical nerve stimulation (TENS)

This technique, based on the gate control theory, is well established in the management of chronic pain. Its role in the management of postoperative pain is less clear because of conflicting data from studies that do not fulfil the necessary criteria for randomised, prospective, double-blind placebo-controlled studies. TENS is non-invasive, non-toxic, continuous, and simple to use. No adverse effects to its use have been reported. Many workers have reported a reduced requirement for opioids in the postoperative period. A reduction in the incidence of postoperative ileus and fewer postoperative pulmonary complications have also been reported. However, no such morphine-sparing effects were seen in other studies. Since TENS produces a distinct tingling sensation, blind, controlled trials are difficult and a placebo effect cannot be ruled out.

Cryoanalgesia

A cryoprobe with its tip chilled to $-60°C$ by liquid nitrogen is applied to the peripheral nerve. Cryolesioning produces a second-degree axonal lesion while preserving the surrounding nerve structure; this allows healing of the nerve without scarring, and consequent recovery of function. Although percutaneous techniques have been described, cryoanaesthesia is usually performed by the surgeon under direct vision. The most common indication is management of pain following thoracotomy. Pain relief may last from weeks to months. There is limited literature on the technique and a lack of controlled studies. Post-thoracotomy analgesia may not be superior to that provided by parenteral morphine. In one study epidural fentanyl infusion was shown to provide better pain relief than cryoanalgesia for post-thoracotomy pain. Complications such as unwanted, prolonged postoperative nipple anaesthesia, skin destruction, chest wall bleeding, and intercostal neuralgia have been described. The possible long-term effects of this technique have not been fully elucidated.

Psychological methods of pain management

Psychological interventions to decrease anxiety about surgery have been used to reduce the postoperative pain experience. Highly beneficial effects of a preoperative informational visit by the anaesthesiologists on post-operative pain, opioid use, and length of hospital stay have been reported.

Deep breathing techniques are used in a variety of clinical situations by most healthcare professionals. Structured deep breathing technique that includes holding the inhalation for several seconds followed by slow complete exhalation slows autonomal arousal and reduces anxiety. Muscle relaxation, alone or combined with imagery and hypnotic techniques, reduces anxiety and pain. Hypnosis is effective for the management of acute pain. The response varies depending on hypnotisability. In susceptible patients, hypnotic suggestion can distract attention from pain for several hours or days. Although hypnosis has many advantages over pharmacological intervention, i.e. reversibility, no drug or equipment cost, no adverse effects, it is not commonly practised. The technique is time consuming, requires the presence of a hypnotist and many training sessions, may not be uniformly effective and sometimes may produce states of anxiety or psychosis. For consistent results, patients need individual training, and follow-up audiotapes alone are rarely effective.

Postoperative pain management in ambulatory surgery

The ever-increasing number of outpatient surgeries creates a demand for anaesthetists to provide the essential features of rapid outpatient recovery—the four "A's" of alertness, analgesia, alimentation, and ambulation. These patients must be capable of going to a medically unsupervised environment without adverse effects such as severe pain, nausea, vomiting, and sedation. Regional anaesthesia, whether by epidural, spinal, or field block techniques, offers a number of advantages to outpatients undergoing surgery. These techniques provide analgesia without sedation, earlier discharge, and prolonged postoperative analgesia. Decreased requirements of intra-muscular opioids reduce the incidence of postoperative nausea. Short-acting local anaesthetic agents (e.g. chloroprocaine, lidocaine, or prilocaine for epidural; lidocaine or procaine for spinal anaesthesia) are appropriate for outpatients. At the end of surgery, wound infiltration with bupivacaine can provide extended postoperative analgesia, so that by the time pain is experienced, it is considerably less severe and usually amenable to oral analgesics. However, not all patients are suitable for regional anaesthesia. Difficulties in performing the block and movement during surgery can be a problem in the very anxious patient. Heavy sedation in such patients may negate the positive aspect of regional anaesthesia.

Oral or rectal administration of potent NSAIDs for the prevention and management of postoperative pain in daycare patients appears to be gaining

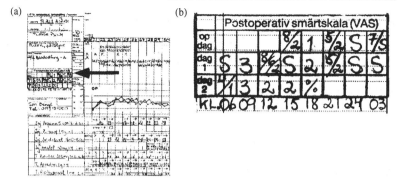

Fig 3.3 (a) Typical bedside vital sign chart in Sweden. To emphasise the importance of regular pain scoring a stamp (arrow) for recording visual analogue scale (VAS) 3 hourly is placed on the space close to the space for recording temperature, pulse, and blood pressure. This facilitates the discussion of postoperative pain on surgical rounds. A pain intensity above 3 on the 10-grade VAS is treated promptly. A glance at the chart will provide information about the adequacy of analgesia and about sleep during the entire treatment period. Easy identification of patients in whom pain is poorly controlled permits prompt revision of management plans. (b) Close-up of the VAS recording stamp. VAS is recorded every 3 hours, it is also recorded before and about 45 minutes after treatment. / = Patient received pain therapy*; for example 8/2 = VAS is 8 before treatment and VAS is 2 after treatment**. S = Patient asleep; ·/· = termination of VAS scoring (when 3 consecutive measurements show VAS ≤ 3 without any treatment); Op dag = operation day (day of surgery); dag 1 = 1 day (after surgery); dag 2 = 2 days; KL = time (clock time). Appropriate modifications are made for daycare surgery patients.

* If VAS > 3 in spite of treatment, a second dose of analgesic (50% of first dose) is given. For example, on day 1 after surgery at 12:00 h pain intensity decreased from 8 to 6 after an injection of analgesic (8/6/2). It decreased to 2 after the second injection. The acute pain nurse or anaesthesiologist is contacted if analgesia is still inadequate after the second injection.

** The dose and route of analgesic are recorded in the nurse report. For patients receiving PCA and spinal opioids respiratory rate, sedation level, and VAS are monitored every hour and documented on a separate paper. (Reproduced from Rawal N, Berggren L. Organization of acute pain services—a low-cost model. *Pain* 1994;57:117–23.)

increasing acceptance. The role of premedication with opioids and NSAIDs and the role of regional block in preventing postoperative pain have been discussed earlier in this chapter.

Organisation of postoperative pain management services

It is increasingly clear that if postoperative analgesia is to be improved on surgical wards, techniques such as PCA, epidural analgesia, and regional blocks have to be used on a routine basis. These techniques provide superior analgesia compared with traditional methods such as intra-

Table 3.12 Organisation of acute pain services at Örebro Medical Centre Hospital, Örebro, Sweden

Healthcare member "pain representatives"	Responsibility
Acute pain anaesthesiologist	Responsible for coordinating hospital-wide acute pain services and in-service teaching
Section anaesthesiologist	Responsible for pre-, peri-, and postoperative care (including postoperative pain) for his/her surgical section
"Pain representative" ward surgeon	Formally responsible for pain management for his/her surgical ward
"Pain representative" day nurse "Pain representative" night nurse	Responsible for implementation of pain management guidelines and monitoring routines on the ward*
Acute pain nurse (nurse anaesthetist)	Daily rounds of all surgical wards
	Check VAS recording on charts (every patient VAS ≤ 3)
	"Trouble-shoot" technical problems (PCA, epidural)
	Refer problem patients to section anaesthesiologist (link between surgical ward and anaesthesiologist)
	Daily "bedside" teaching of ward nurses

* Patients are treated on the basis of standard orders and protocols developed jointly by chiefs of anaesthesiology, surgery, and nursing sections. Pain representatives meet every 3 months to discuss and implement improvements in surgical ward pain management routines.

Note: This organisation benefits about 20 000 patients a year (VAS ≤ 3), it has been functioning satisfactorily since 1991. Cost per patient is US $2–3.

muscular opioids but have their own risks and therefore require special monitoring. Traditional methods are not risk free either but risks have not been quantified. While better pain relief is relatively easily achievable, there has to be a balance between acceptable risk, perceived benefit, and cost-effectiveness. Without an effective organisation on surgical wards, pain management will remain unsatisfactory. National interdisciplinary expert committee reports from Australia,[20] the UK,[21] the USA[22], and from the International Association for Study of Pain (IASP)[23] have recommended the establishment of acute pain services (APS) based on a team approach (anaesthesiologists, surgeons, ward nurses) to improve pain management. APS models developed in different countries and institutions may vary considerably because of differences in healthcare systems, nursing regulations, fund allocations, and availability of equipment and personnel.

In the USA, comprehensive pain management teams consisting of staff anaesthetists, resident anaesthetists, specially trained nurses, and pharmacists have been available for a decade. These APS have had a considerable impact on increasing the awareness of the problem of postoperative pain. However, these anaesthetist-based APS benefit selected patients (at best less than 10–15% of the surgical population) and are too expensive (US $100–300 per patient). Simpler and less expensive APS models have to be

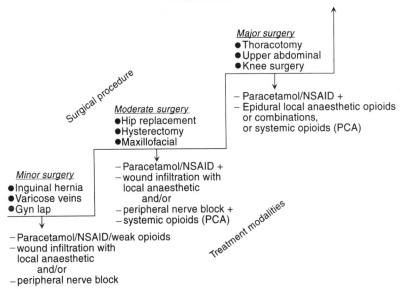

Fig 3.4   Analgesia ladder for postoperative pain. Frequent pain assessment and its documentation on the patient chart will improve pain management. This can be greatly facilitated by an organised pain service which includes anaesthesiologists, surgeons, and ward nurses. (Gyn lap = gynaecological laparotomy; NSAID = non-steroidal anti-inflammatory drugs. (Developed jointly by Jørgen Dahl, Denmark and Narinder Rawal, Sweden)

developed if the aim is to improve the quality of postoperative analgesia for every patient who undergoes surgery, whether it is inpatient or ambulatory. Furthermore, quality assurance measures such as frequent assessment and documentation of pain can no longer be ignored.

A low-cost nurse-based anaesthetist-supervised APS for every patient who undergoes surgery at our hospital (about 20 000 patients a year) has been described. The cornerstone of our APS is pain assessment and documentation on vital sign chart by trained ward nurses, which is done every 3 hours for inpatients and every hour for outpatients (Fig 3.3).[24]

The goal of pain management is that no patient should have a VAS score greater than 3 (of 10) during rest or movement. Patient treatment is based on standard orders and protocols developed by anaesthesiology, surgery, and nursing sections. An acute pain nurse (APN) provides an effective link between the three disciplines (Table 3.12). Ward nurse and surgeon participation are crucial in this organisation. Another critical element to improving pain management is the development of protocols and training of ward nurses.

Routine recording of pain scores has underscored that a VAS less than 3 frequently cannot be maintained with intramuscular opioids in patients with severe pain, such as those undergoing thoracic upper abdominal or major knee surgery. In such patients postoperative analgesia is provided by epidural local anaesthetics and/or opioids. A "ladder" has been proposed for postoperative pain which is similar to the "WHO ladder" for the management of cancer pain (Fig 3.4). It is important to remember that a majority of patients (80–90%) do not require epidural analgesia or PCA. At our hospital titrated intravenous opioid dosing is replacing intramuscular injection on a hospital-wide basis as the routine pain management therapy. The additional cost of our nurse-based APS is the salary of 1·5 APN, which averages out at $2–3 per patient.

Summary

The prevention, recognition, and management of postoperative pain in adults, as well as in children, has been receiving a great deal of interest lately. In spite of advances in the understanding of the pathophysiology of acute pain and the neural pathways that transmit nociception, and in the development of new analgesic medications and drug delivery techniques, many patients continue to suffer from unrelieved acute pain. The poor outcome obtained with current regimens is primarily due to the inadequacies of drug administration techniques and lack of pain scoring routines, rather than the qualities of opioids themselves.

The choice of postoperative pain management depends on the site of surgery, technique and equipment availability, monitoring facilities, and the expertise of the patient's physicians. The technique of postoperative analgesia may have a significant influence on several aspects of recovery. Although it is well recognised that pain management by intermittent injection of opioids is woefully inadequate, most patients continue to receive intramuscular opioids because of the simplicity of, and familiarity with, this technique. However, the introduction of simple methods of pain scoring and a greater degree of flexibility in the administration of opioids would lead to considerable improvement in the management of postoperative pain.

The efficacious treatment of acute postoperative pain and post-traumatic pain is seriously deficient in modern health care. Effective means of controlling acute pain are available. Psychological effects of acute pain need to be understood and non-pharmacological interventions employed when indicated. Patients need to be taught that they can expect and have the right to have their pain relieved. Many of the drugs and drug delivery systems have been available for years and their present underutilisation may be a reflection of the lack of emphasis on the importance of management of acute pain. Certain techniques such as epidural local anaesthetic infusions and spinal opioids require specialised monitoring. Other techniques such as the infiltration of a wound with local anaesthetic or addition of NSAIDs to oral opioids are so simple that excluding them from patient care is almost callous and inconsiderate. With well-organised clinical services established to provide modern analgesia, the risks associated with epidural opioids, PCA, and other modern techniques may be no higher than with intramuscular opioid injections. Careful patient selection, appropriate choice of drugs and dosage, nurse education, and adequate supervision can result in the safe application of all these methods.

References

1 Marks RM, Sachar EJ. Undertreatment of medical inpatients with narcotic analgesics. *Ann Intern Med* 1973;**78**:172–81.
2 Utting JE, Smith JM. Postoperative analgesia. *Anaesthesia* 1979;**34**:320–32.
3 Oden RV. Acute postoperative pain: incidence, severity, and the etiology of inadequate treatment. *Anaesth Clin North Am* 1989;**7**:1–17.
4 Warfield CA, Kahn CH. Acute pain management. Programs in US hospitals and experiences and attitudes among US adults. *Anesthesiology* 1995;**83**:1090–4.
5 Rawal N. Acute pain services in Europe—a 17-nation survey. *Reg Anesth* 1995;**20**:A85.
6 Rawal N, Sjöstrand U, Christoffersson E, *et al.* Comparison of intramuscular and epidural morphine for postoperative analgesia in the grossly obese: influence on postoperative ambulation and pulmonary function. *Anesth Analg* 1984;**63**:583–92.
7 Blomberg S, Emanuelsson H, Ricksten SE. Thoracic epidural anesthesia and central hemodynamics in patients with unstable angina pectoris. *Anesth Analg* 1989;**69**:558–62.
8 Lavies N, Hart L, Rounsefell B, Runeiman W. Identification of patient, medical and nursing staff attitudes to postoperative opioid analgesia: stage I of a longitudinal study of postoperative analgesia. *Pain* 1992;**48**:313–9.
9 Cohen FL. Postsurgical pain relief: patients' status and nurses' medication choices. *Pain* 1980;**9**:265–74.
10 McQuay H. Pre-emptive analgesia: a systematic review of clinical studies. *Ann Med* 1995;**27**:249–56.
11 Breivik H. Pre-emptive analgesia. *Curr Opin Anaesthesiol* 1994;**7**:458–61.
12 Rosow C. Agonist–antagonist opioids: theory and clinical practice. *Can J Anaesth* 1989;**36**;S5–8.
13 Björkman R. Central antinociceptive effects of non-steroidal anti-inflammatory drugs and paracetamol—experimental studies in the rat. *Acta Anaesthesiol Scand* 1995;**39**:3–44.
14 Sechzer PH, Wachtel J, Keats AS. Circulatory lability and myocardial stress in patients undergoing cardiovascular surgery. *Am J Surg* 1968;**116**:683–92.
15 Rawal N. Patient-controlled analgesia (PCA) for postoperative pain—a European survey. *Reg Anesth* 1995;**20**:A134.
16 Eisenach JC, Lysak SZ, Viscomi CM. Epidural clonidine analgesia following surgery. *Anesthesiology* 1989;**71**:640–6.
17 Wang KH, Nauss LA, Thomas JE. Pain relief by intrathecally applied morphine in man. *Anesthesiology* 1979;**50**:149–51.
18 Behar M, Magora F, Olshwang D, Davidson JT. Epidural morphine in treatment of pain. *Lancet* 1979;**i**:527–8.
19 Rawal N, Hylander J, Allvin R, *et al.* Postoperative patient-controlled regional analgesia at home. *Reg Anesth* 1997;**22**:S82.
20 National Health and Medical Research Council (Australia). *Management of severe pain.* Canberra, Australia, 1988.
21 Royal College of Surgeons of England and the College of Anaesthetists. *Report of the Working Party on Pain after Surgery,* September, 1990.
22 US Department of Health and Human Services. *Acute pain management. Clinical practice guidelines.* AHCPR Publications No. 92–0032, USA, 1992.
23 International Association for the Study (IASP). Management of acute pain. In: Ready LB, Edwards WT, eds., *A practical guide task force on acute pain.* IASP Publications, 1992.

24 Rawal N, Berggren L. Organization of acute pain services—a low-cost model. *Pain* 1994;**57**:117–23.

Selected reading

Black AMS. Taking pains to take away pain. Time for hospitals to set up an acute pain service (Editorial). *BMJ* 1991;**302**:1165–6.

Brevik H, ed. Postoperative pain management. *Baillière's Clin Anaesthesiol* 1995;**9**:403–585.

Macintyre PE, Ready LB. *Acute pain management. A practical guide.* London: WB Saunders, 1996.

Rawal N. Neuraxial administration of opioids and nonopioids. In: Brown D, ed., *Regional anesthesia and analgesia.* Philadelphia: WB Saunders, 1996:208–31.

Ready LB, Rawal N. Anesthesiology-based acute pain services. A contemporary view. In: Brown D, ed., *Regional anesthesia and analgesia.* Philadelphia: WB Saunders, 1996:632–43.

Sandler AN. Current concepts in acute pain control. *Anaesthesiol Clin N Am* 1992;**10**:211–451.

4: Obstetric pain management

ANDRÉ VAN ZUNDERT

History of pain relief in childbirth

Methods of pain relief during childbirth were described in ancient writings. Opiates and soporifics were employed in China, wine and brandy in European countries. Substances such as mandragora, hemp, poppy, hemlock and hyascyamus were mixed and boiled and then applied, swallowed or inhaled from a sponge.

The techniques used in obstetric anaesthesia and analgesia are the same as in surgery, although the historical development of pain relief in childbirth is influenced by folklore and superstition, while medical and religious objections delayed their application in labour. Modern obstetric analgesia was initially used in 1847 by James Young Simpson from Edinburgh, who was the first person to use ether and later chloroform anaesthesia in obstetrics. "Sleep has stopped the pains", described the patients afterwards. Simpson had to defend the concept of pain relief during labour constantly, but the turning point occurred in 1853 when chloroform was administered to Queen Victoria for the delivery of Prince Leopold. Other inhalation anaesthetics were discovered, for instance cyclopropane and ethylene-oxygen. These became very popular in some centres, although expensive and complicated apparatus were necessary, with the constant presence of a physician. In 1853 it became clear that chloroform anaesthesia affected the fetus by transplacental transfer. Later ether was also instilled rectally as a liquid. A first-line method of pain relief in labour is a mixture of 50% nitrous oxide and 50% oxygen (Entonox), which is still very popular today. Morphine injections to control labour pain were initiated in the last century, although the "respiratory injury" to the child restricted their use. Scopolamine, producing "twilight sleep", caused fetal and neonatal asphyxia and adverse effects on the uterine contractions. All newer opioids, such as pethidine, butorphanol, nalbuphine, and pentazocine, also caused neonatal depression. Tranquillisers, barbiturates, and sedatives were introduced, as it was hoped that these drugs would allow reduction in the dose of the opioid, and would result in less depression of the fetal respiratory centre than opioids. Many workers realised that the effect on the child of a drug given to the mother is directly proportional to the amount given and the duration of its action. In the 1950s, "natural childbirth" became quite popular in Europe. In fact, the Dick-Read method ("Natural childbirth" and "Childbirth without fear") and the "Psychoprophylactic method" of Lamaze in France failed to produce a painless delivery. Acupuncture and transcutaneous electrical nerve stimulation, applied during labour, also resulted in incomplete analgesia.

Regional anaesthesia using local anaesthetics was preferable to inhalational anaesthesia because pain relief was similar, with less side-effects such as vomiting. Oskar Kreis was the first to use spinal anaesthesia with cocaine for operative vaginal delivery in 1900 in Basle, Switzerland. Pudendal and paracervical nerve block were propagated in the first half of this century, although the high incidence of fetal distress secondary to the uptake of local anaesthetic and uterine hypertonus led to an almost abandonment of paracervical blocks. Von Stoeckel, in 1909, was the first to use procaine via the caudal route in order to relieve labour pain. Unless large doses were used, caudal anaesthesia did not relieve the pain of uterine contractions. This approach inevitably resulted in problems of toxic effects and retardation of labour. The lumbar epidural approach was described by the Spanish military surgeon Pagès in 1921, and later Dogliotti described the loss-of-resistance technique for epidural anaesthesia. The introduction in 1949 of lidocaine (three times as active, less toxic and longer acting than procaine) and in 1963 bupivacaine (longer acting, although more toxic) became major factors in promoting the use of continuous epidural analgesia for labour pain.[1] Labour could be pain free from start to finish, without the need for any pharmacological depression of the fetus or neonate. Jouppila and his Finnish colleagues demonstrated that, using radioacive xenon to measure the placental blood flow, epidural analgesia results in no change or even an improvement in the intervillous blood flow.[2] Epidural analgesia still has its undesirable effects, including reducing the efficiency of uterine contractions and weakening the abdominal muscles, which lead to less expulsion forces and delayed second stages with more instrumental deliveries.

The nature of pain in parturition

The Rumanian Aburel demonstrated in 1930 the afferent fibres carrying pain impulses from the uterus to a plexus lying in the angle between the aorta and the vertebral column.[3] Later Cleland and Bonica confirmed these by extensive anatomical dissections.[4][5] Pain in the first stage of labour primarily results from dilatation of the cervix and lower uterine segment and from distention of the body of the uterus by uterine contractions.

90

Nerve fibres transmitting pain sensation during the first stage of labour travel with sympathetic fibres and enter the neuraxis at the tenth, eleventh, and twelfth thoracic and first lumbar spinal segments (see Fig. 4.1). In addition to the pain of contraction, descent of the fetal head into the pelvis causes distention of the pelvic structures and pressure on roots of the lumbosacral plexus. Pain produced by stretching of the perineum is transmitted by the pudendal nerve, which is derived from the second, third and fourth sacral nerves. However, long before the descent of the fetal head into the pelvis and the stretching of the perineum, in a number of women labour pain cannot be successfully relieved without anaesthetising the sacral roots. Persistent posterior position of the presenting part or dystocia is the reason, according to Bonica.[5] Beside neural and biochemical mechanisms that participate in the modulation of nociception, the individual's total pain experience is also influenced by motivational, affective, cognitive, emotional and psychological factors, the environment and personality of the mother, as well as ethnic and cultural factors.

A lot of misconceptions and confusions have been made about the nature of the pain during childbirth. In primitive societies in Australia and Africa, most parturients manifested severe pain behaviour.[6] A study by Lefèbre and Carli of parturition in 88 individuals of 29 species of captive and wild non-human primates revealed that 78% manifested moderate to very severe

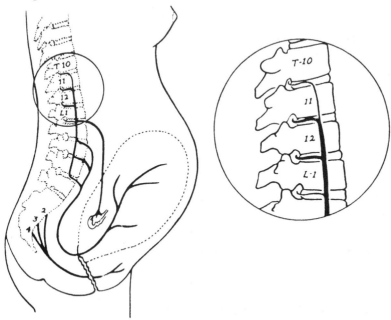

Fig 4.1   Parturition pain pathways. Reproduced with permission from Bonica JJ. *The management of pain*, 2nd edn. Philadelphia: Lea and Febiger, 1990

pain, characterised by straining, stretching, arching, grimacing, writhing, shaking, restlessness, and vocalisations.[7] Swedish investigators found that the prevalence of intolerable severe pain ranged from 35 to 58%,[8] and 77% of primiparae reported that pain during childbirth was severe or intolerable. Bonica studied in 121 obstetric centres (with some having 100–150 deliveries daily) in 35 countries on six continents the frequency and intensity of labour pain and found that 15% had little or no pain, 35% had moderate pain, 30% had severe pain, and 20% had extremely severe pain during parturition.[6] Melzack noted that the pain rating index scores for labour pain were some 8–10 points higher than those associated with back pain, cancer pain, phantom limb pain, or postherpetic neuralgia, and even greater than acute pain that occurs after accidents.[9]

Adverse effects of labour pain on the fetus

Although it is known that analgesic drugs during labour and delivery are potentially dangerous to mother and fetus, skilful administration may offer fetal and neonatal benefits. Analgesic drugs may act therapeutically by increasing the oxygen supply to the fetus and diminishing maternal sympathetic nervous system activity. This results in an improved uterine blood flow.[10]

Indications for regional anaesthesia in obstetrics

The goals of pain relief during anaesthesia for obstetrics are to provide effective and safe pain relief during the first, second and third stages of labour and delivery without interfering with the process of labour and delivery, to minimise the side-effects for the mother and the fetus and, finally, to improve maternal satisfaction.

Epidural analgesia gives major advantages in parturients presenting with pregnancy-induced hypertension (PIH) and pre-eclampsia. It also provides better pain relief and stress management, easier control of maternal blood pressure, and if in place it is available for assisted delivery should the maternal or fetal condition deteriorate. These patients can present with severe haemodynamic derangements. Severe PIH associated with thrombocytopenia and elevated liver enzymes—the HELLP syndrome (haemolysis, elevated liver enzymes, low platelets)—has a high mortality rate and requires intensive care treatment. Monitoring is essential in these patients, and this includes invasive haemodynamic monitoring, with pulmonary artery pressure and intra-arterial pressure monitoring, especially during an anaesthetic or when intravenous venodilators such as sodium nitroprusside are used.

Special consideration should be given to parturients presenting with diseases of major organs (e.g. cardiac, respiratory, liver, renal disease, diabetes). Each disease adapts to pregnancy through different mechanisms, and changes in the equilibrium between the pulmonary and systemic circulation induced by stress and/or disease of the woman. The anaesthetist should be informed thoroughly about any problems that may be encountered in the patient, so that the decision whether or not to give regional anaesthesia can be taken. The disease may have an effect on the pregnancy and vice versa. The disease can also worsen during pregnancy.

Abnormal presentations (e.g. brow/face/shoulder/breech presentations, umbilical cord prolapse, multiple gestation) are often a challenge for the obstetric team. Close communication between the obstetrician and anaesthetist regarding the anaesthetic plan provides the optimal outcome. Lumbar epidural anaesthesia is recommended for labour analgesia and delivery, as often a trial of labour may result in the need for a caesarean delivery. One should anticipate and be prepared for the rapidly changing obstetric and anaesthetic needs of these parturients.

Contraindications for the use of regional anaesthesia in obstetrics

Placental abruption and placenta previa are the commonest causes of antepartum haemorrhage. If bleeding is severe or a coagulopathy supervenes, major regional anaesthesia is contraindicated. Rupture of the uterus is an uncommon but potentially lethal complication of labour and delivery. Emergency caesarean deliveries under general anaesthesia are often the only choice for the above.

Epidural technique for vaginal deliveries

While some anaesthetists perform an epidural standing, the seated position is more comfortable, steadies movements, and brings the eye much nearer to the field of operation.[11] The back is aseptically prepared and covered with sterile drapes. The entry is fixed by placing two fingers on either side of the interspace selected and a small amount of local anaesthetic (e.g. lidocaine 1–2%) is infiltrated into the subcutaneous tissues. Under aseptic conditions a 16- to 18-gauge epidural Tuohy needle is inserted using the midline position, usually in the L2–3, L3–4 or L4–5 interspace.

The epidural space is usually identified by the Dogliotti loss-of-resistance technique with saline as the seeker solution, although some prefer to use air. The loss-of-resistance method gives tactile evidence of entry into the epidural space. The needle is inserted in a rather cranial and strictly median direction and is advanced with a smooth, continuous motion. Further movement of the needle is halted when the resistance of the ligamentum flavum changes. The anaesthetist's thumb exerts continuous positive pressure on the end of the piston of the syringe, until sudden loss of resistance indicates that the advancing needle point leaves the ligamentum flavum and enters the epidural space.[12]

The hanging-drop technique is an alternative, which gives visual identification, but will result in more accidental dura punctures, depending on the skills of the anaesthetist. A clear nylon 60 cm catheter with a closed-end top with three marginal openings (helical eyes) and markings and with a detachable luer fitting is used. The catheter should not meet resistance when advanced, otherwise it should be replaced. Complaints about pain or paraesthesia in the left or right leg are considered to indicate that the catheter is situated too far to the left or to the right. If this is the case, the Tuohy needle must be replaced. Attempts to advance the catheter when an elastic resistance is felt may result in venepuncture. If the catheter enters a vein several times, another puncture is made one segment higher or lower. Whenever an additional injection is given, one should always bear in mind that an originally correctly situated catheter may take an intrathecal or intravenous position.[13] This is one of the many reasons why one should not, under any circumstances, inject rapidly and always attempt to adhere to minimum doses. The catheter is advanced cranially to the level where the 20 cm marking disappears into the needle. Only after the Tuohy needle has been removed, the catheter is pulled back until 3 cm lies within the epidural space. To keep it deeper is of little use, hampers the induction of perineal analgesia and enhances the risk of unilateral analgesia. To recognise a possible intrathecal or intravenous position, carefully and progressively aspirate through the catheter with a well-fitting 5 ml syringe. From the insertion point at the skin, the first 3 cm of the catheter are directed away from the midline to prevent compression by the spine. The site of the puncture and the catheter are taped to the back with adhesive plaster.

Repeated changing of syringes remains the greatest problem in maintaining sterility. An antibacterial filter also prevents the injection of particulate matter such as glass or rubber. It should be borne in mind that aspirating through a filter is clearly more difficult. Identify clearly the epidural tubing in order to avoid any unwanted injection. The patient is then placed in a semi-sitting position with a wedge under the right hip to displace the uterus to the left. A well-placed catheter holds the promise of smooth anaesthesia, while a dubiously placed catheter means a dubious prognosis for the coming hours. In case of doubt, it is therefore appropriate to reposition the catheter until it is correctly situated. The extra work may save the patient, and the anaesthetist, from any inconvenience.

If the aspiration test results in the return of CSF, another interspace should be chosen for a repeat attempt to place the needle in the epidural space, or in the case of caesarean deliveries, the subarachnoid space should be used to institute spinal anaesthesia. If the aspiration test yields a bloody return, it is probable that one of the veins of the epidural plexus has been punctured. Another interspace should be chosen for a repeat attempt to place the needle in the epidural space. Injection of a small amount of local anaesthetic, e.g. 3 ml of a local anaesthetic solution (bupivacaine 0·5% or lidocaine 2%), should not result in any major anaesthetic effect if the needle is in the epidural space. However, if the dura has been pierced and the local anaesthetic is injected into the subarachnoid space, extensive sensory and motor block may be noted, depending on the dose of local anaesthetic given. Large amounts of local anaesthetics for epidural anaesthesia should not be given as a bolus, but should be divided in small incremental or fractional (3–5 ml) doses at intervals of at least 60 seconds, until the total dose given for a single-dose epidural block has been administered, while at the same time the patient is monitored (e.g. vital signs, blood pressure, spread of anaesthesia, sensory and motor blockade).[14] With the patient resting comfortably, the spread of sensory anaesthesia is checked frequently by gentle repeated pinpricks or by a cotton swab moistened with alcohol, with the latter being more pleasant for the woman. If the intermittent technique is used, appropriate top-up doses can be given on a regular basis as needed by the patient. Alternatively, a continuous infusion of local anaesthetic with or without opioids can be given. For labour and vaginal delivery, all local anaesthetics (e.g. chloroprocaine, lidocaine and bupivacaine in a variety of concentrations, with or without epinephrine or opioids) have been used. By using a low concentration of bupivacaine in a rather large volume (10 ml), most of the potential objections to the use of epidural analgesia in childbirth can be overcome. Epidural analgesia using bupivacaine 0·125% plus adrenaline 1:800 000 is effective and safe for the control of pain during vaginal delivery. It provides effective analgesia during labour and delivery and it even allows postpartum examination of the uterus and perineal repair, if necessary, without the need for any other anaesthetic intervention. This dosage causes minimal or no motor block, does not lead to a prolonged expulsion time, not even in breech deliveries, and the maternal and neonatal plasma concentrations are well below the toxic level.[16] By adding sufentanil 5–10 mg to the above mentioned 10 ml solution, Vertommen et al. found, in a multicentre study, that the duration of analgesia was longer and the quality of analgesia could be improved from 92% (no sufentanil) to 99% (sufentanil), while the total dose of bupivacaine was significantly less (34 vs 42 mg), and the instrumental delivery rate was also significantly lower (24% vs 36%).[17] This study proved that variations in the epidural solution can reduce the incidence of instrumental deliveries, by using minute doses of local anaesthetics (thereby avoiding or minimising motor block) combined with small amounts of opioids. This brings us close to the ideal analgesic method, on the one hand providing effective maternal analgesia during labour and delivery and, on the other hand, avoiding the negative effects on the mother and the fetus of interfering with the progress of labour.

Epidural analgesia for labour and delivery differs considerably from operative epidural analgesia technique and postoperative epidural analgesia. In obstetrics, the aim is selective analgesia, with minimal influence on muscle power and duration of labour, and with the lowest toxicity for the mother and the fetus. Fortunately, the pain of normal uterine contractions seems to be more readily relieved than pathological pain. This is an important factor because it allows the use of low concentrations of local anaesthetic and minimal doses of opioids. A second important factor is the fact that the intensity and the site of analgesia vary considerably not only between parturients, but also during the course of labour in the same individual. The intermittent technique provides the optimal goals of obstetric analgesia for vaginal delivery—for each top-up the appropriate time, dose and position can be chosen, thus flattening the "peak and valleys" to produce a true continuous analgesia, provided an anaesthetist is immediately available at the labour ward. Bupivacaine 0·125% plus adrenaline 1:800 000, combined with or preceded by sufentanil, is effective and safe for epidural use in vaginal deliveries. To obtain 20 ml of this solution mix 5 ml of the commercially available bupivacaine 0·5% plus adrenaline 1:200 000 with 15 ml of sterile physiological saline without preservative. To this 20 ml is added 0·4 ml of sufentanil 50 mg/ml to give a 1 mg/ml solution of sufentanil.

Start of epidural analgesia

Analgesia is induced when the obstetrician judges that labour is established, and the woman asks for pain relief, regardless of the degree of dilatation.

Monitoring of the obstetric patient

A careful check-up is ideally performed in the weeks prior to delivery in a non-hurried situation, where the woman also receives information. In some countries this is performed by obstetric staff where the anaesthetist is involved to check it is necessary only to see the patient's notes for the medical and surgical history, and what kind of drugs are to be given.

Inspection of the patient's back is essential and this is best performed in a non-stressful situation. In the labour ward, she is monitored for uterine contractions, blood pressure and fetal heart rate, while an infusion is running prior to the block.[18] To optimise patient safety when epidural and/or subarachnoid local anaesthetics and opioids are used, the monitoring needs to be considered. Observation of respiratory rate and mental status by trained personnel is the optimal monitoring technique but too labour intensive and therefore not cost effective. Even with observation of the respiratory rate, tidal volume may be diminished, resulting in hypercapnia.

Current monitoring technologies include impedance apnoea monitoring, pulse oximetry, capnography, and arterial blood gas analysis. While capnography may be the most sensitive, non-intubated patients find a tight-fitting mask uncomfortable, while with a mask that is not properly fitted, capnography is unreliable. Pulse oximetry is a reliable method of monitoring oxygen delivery to the peripheral tissues, is easy to use, less expensive, and readily accepted by patients. Its one drawback is that it does not provide information on increasing P_{CO_2} levels.

Making the parturient pain free

What drug and how much will be given as a loading dose depends on the severity of pain and also largely on the degree of dilatation and the expected duration and progress of labour.

Normal, well-established labour

Although most departments will have "treatment guidelines" and "standard" doses, many parturients will not receive a "standard" treatment because there are so many variables in labour, both in the experience of pain and in the response to treatment. Moderate pain will be treated more aggressively in a more advanced stage of labour than the same degree of pain at an early stage. The onset of labour is also more gradual when induced with oxytocin than with prostaglandin, and pain tends to increase more sharply with prostaglandin. The "normal" first dose is 10 ml of bupivacaine 0·125% plus adrenaline 1:800 000 plus sufentanil 1:1 000 000, i.e. 12·5 mg of bupivacaine plus 12·5 μg of adrenaline plus 10 μg of sufentanil injected over approximately 45 seconds. Blood pressure is measured every minute for the first 10 minutes and at 5-minute intervals thereafter. If the woman starts yawning, looks pale, feels drowsy or vomits, aortocaval compression is suspected and treated by increasing left uterine displacement. After 10 minutes most parturients will have substantial pain relief, but it will take another 10 minutes before meaningful testing by cold or pinprick can be done, although full extension of skin anaesthesia will take even more time. Motor block should be tested earlier, especially when pain relief is fast and complete. If the motor block on the Bromage scale is 66% or 100%, subarachnoid placement of the catheter is most likely. If this situation is confirmed by the appropriate tests, the catheter is left in place. When a top-up is needed, 4 ml of the starting solution is given. If after 15 minutes there is little or no pain relief, the possibility of intravascular placement of the epidural catheter has to be considered. Remove the bacterial filter and aspirate with a 2 ml syringe. If negative, connect the parturient to an ECG monitor or the plethysmograph of an oximeter, or use the direct ECG mode of the fetal monitor. Also apply an automatic non-invasive blood pressure monitor, if not already in use. Explain to the parturient the possible signs of intravenous adrenaline and local anaesthetic, such as palpitations, headache, change in taste, or tinnitus. Then

97

inject again, over 40 seconds, 10 ml of bupivacaine 0·125% plus adrenaline 12·5 μg plus sufentanil 10 μg. If there are no signs or symptoms of intravenous placement of the catheter, wait another 15 minutes for pain relief. If there is none, replace the catheter and restart the procedure. As it is not yet known what is the safe dose of sufentanil given in a short time, the maximum dose is 30 μg. Further studies are warranted to find the optimum dose of sufentanil to be added to the solution, as sufentanil 5 μg seems to give the same results as 7·5 or 10 μg.

Very advanced or rapidly progressing labour

Rapid treatment of the already considerable pain is essential, since the pain of the second stage may come before or shortly after the pain of the first stage is controlled. When the anaesthetist is asked for an epidural anaesthetic in far advanced labour, it may be better to opt for spinal anaesthesia or a sequential spinal-epidural analgesia using very fine long spinal needles through a Tuohy needle, which is placed in the epidural space. When the long spinal needle is in the subarachnoid space, the local anaesthetic can be injected in order to produce a subarachnoid block with a fast onset (e.g. 1 ml bupivacaine 0·5% plus 5 μg sufentanil). Then the long spinal needle is removed and an epidural catheter is introduced through the Tuohy needle into the epidural space, which allows the usual epidural top-ups to be given when necessary.

If only the epidural technique is used, the first dose will be 14 ml of bupivacaine 0·125% plus adrenaline 1:800 000 plus sufentanil 1:1 000 000. If it is necessary to provide pain relief rapidly by the epidural route or when insertion of the catheter does not go smoothly or proves to be difficult, this first dose can be given through the needle as the situation allows, and a catheter is inserted afterwards. During this time, the pregnant woman is observed closely because if this dose enters the subarachnoid space the result will be a surgical spinal anaesthesia requiring a larger fluid infusion and probably a vasopressor such as ephedrine. If pain relief is still insufficient after 15 minutes, it is wise to make sure by questioning and vaginal examination that the beginning of the second stage is not the origin of pain. A second dose will be given, but if the second stage has started it should be given in the sitting position. If this second dose does not result in a pain-free patient after 10 minutes, go through the list of possible reasons for persisting pain: full bladder, full dilatation, scar dehiscence after previous caesarean delivery, wrong position of the catheter. If the catheter is wrongly placed, a new one should be inserted if time allows.

Very early painful labour

Sometimes an obstetrician will ask for pain relief in a patient who, in very early labour, already complains of serious discomfort. At this very early stage, 10 ml of the solution described above may stop the contractions for some time. A reassuring talk with the patient, promising that everything is prepared to provide analgesia if the pain gets worse, and installing the catheter, will often help. If this is not enough, most women can be made comfortable without interference with labour by the epidural administration of 10 ml of sufentanil 1 : 1 000 000. Depending on the evolution of labour, this may be repeated a second time before switching to the usual local anaesthetic plus opioid. It should be kept in mind that 10 μg of sufentanil is not suitable as a test dose. The effects (pain relief) or side-effects (drowsiness, vomiting, respiratory depression, pruritus) of an unintentional intravenous injection will be weak or unobserved.

The maintenance dose: keeping the parturient pain free

Once good analgesia has been achieved everything becomes easier: the effect of the doses becomes more predictable and the results more reliable. What is not known in advance is when the maintenance doses will be needed. On average, 10 ml of bupivacaine 0·125% plus adrenaline 1 : 800 000 will produce analgesia for about 1 hour, whereas the same dose including 10 μg of sufentanil will work for about 1.5 hours. When giving the top-up dose, this is the time to ask the midwife or the obstetrician about the evolution of labour. In this way the return of pain can be anticipated and analgesia adapted to the progress of labour with the standard 10 ml solution, until a total dose of 30 μg of sufentanil has been administered. There are a number of reasons for giving a top-up to a pain-free parturient. It is better to prevent pain than to relieve pain. When using a low dose–low concentration technique, the effect of the local anaesthetic will wear off rather quickly. If one waits too long, anaesthesia can be gone completely, and one has to start all over again. More prolonged labours provide the opportunity to learn how long a dose works in one particular individual. On a busy obstetric ward, it is preferable to give the occasional top-up dose in advance when the anaesthetist is free, rather than risk having to attend three or more parturients at the same time. With low doses, it is better to inject too early rather than too late because of the mild influence on sympathetic and motor block. Another reason for a top-up dose is the demand for block of the sacral segments because of complaints of perineal pain or when the expulsion of the fetus is expected.

In summary, there are three reasons for injecting the epidural dose for a parturient:

1 The induction dose
2 The prevention of pain when it becomes apparent that the previous dose is wearing off
3 The need for perineal analgesia if not already present.

Waiting to give the top-up dose until the pain returns, results in the typical "peak and valley" method. A pain-free labour and delivery is preferable to some pain-free intervals. The mother will lose confidence in our ability to control her pain and it may take considerable time and effort to re-establish good analgesia once it is lost. The mother is asked to warn the anaesthetist when awareness of still pain-free contractions returns. That is about the time for a top-up.

Alternative techniques

Continuous epidural infusion technique

Continuous epidural infusion of local anaesthetic became popular some 15 years ago in the hope of avoiding fluctuation in the quality of pain relief and worse, and to avoid situations where a patient loses analgesia altogether. In the latter case, the patient may experience severe pain before the anaesthetist can re-establish pain relief. Continuous epidural infusion decreases the requirement for bolus injections during labour, and it also decreases the requirement for administration of local anaesthetic just before delivery. This is advantageous on a busy obstetric service, where the anaesthetist may not always be able to provide additional bolus injections of local anaesthetic on demand. The anaesthetist only starts the continuous epidural infusion until satisfactory sensory anaesthesia has been established by performing bolus injection of a local anaesthetic. By avoiding fluctuation in the extent of sympathetic blockade, the continuous epidural infusion technique reduces the risk of hypotension. Another advantage of the continuous technique is clear in the case of migration of an initially satisfactorily positioned catheter into an epidural vein. If this should occur during continuous infusion, there would be a slow intravenous infusion of local anaesthetic, which initially should not cause systemic toxicity. Recession of the level of sensory anaesthesia would represent evidence of intravenous administration of local anaesthetic. However, the use of the continuous epidural infusion technique will not prevent the intravenous injection of local anaesthetic during induction or maintenance of epidural anaesthesia.

The reported total doses of bupivacaine received by the continuous-infusion group are more than in the intermittent bolus group, although no dangerous accumulation of local anaesthetic in mother or fetus has been demonstrated. As a consequence, a higher incidence of leg weakness is found in the continuous-infusion group. As there is less manipulation of the epidural catheter, the continuous-infusion technique might decrease the risk of infection. This technique is also very convenient in clinical practice, although careful observation of the parturient should be the same as with the use of the intermittent technique. The continuous technique will not prevent unintentional venous or dural punctures, although these complications usually occur with initial placement of the catheter. Providing epidural anaesthesia to an obstetric patient is the same as giving "tailored anaesthesia", just enough to do the job in this particular case and situation, which can vary from one parturient to another and in a particular parturient it may vary from moment to moment. Therefore individualisation of the pain management is necessary. If anaesthetists try to eliminate the need for "top-up" injections, they will give some patients more local anaesthetic than they need.

In the continuous-infusion technique, patient management should be individualised, just as it should be with the intermittent epidural bolus technique. Accurate and reliable infusion pumps are necessary if the continuous-infusion technique is used and adjustment should be possible. Clearly labelled pumps (avoiding other "unintentional" injections) with a back-up power source (to be used in the event of a power failure) and a written protocol, containing strict rules regarding use of the continuous epidural infusion pumps, are required.

Although chloroprocaine is also used extensively in the intermittent technique, bupivacaine has emerged as the most popular local anaesthetic for obstetric epidural analgesia provided with the intermittent and the continuous-infusion technique. The same solution as above (bupivacaine 0·125% plus adrenaline 1:800 000 plus sufentanil 1:1 000 000) can be used in the continuous-infusion technique at a rate of 6–8 ml/h, starting 45–60 minutes after giving the usual 10 ml bolus dose of the same solution, if this resulted in good analgesia without untoward effects. PCA and PCEA also can provide excellent pain relief for labour, with the potential for utilisation of lower amounts of local anaesthetics, although a clear interaction should exist between parturient and anaesthetist. Perhaps ropivacaine, with less cardiotoxic effects and less motor blockade, may, in the future, prove to give better results in obstetrics.

Combined spinal-epidural anaesthesia technique

Although epidural and spinal anaesthetics are well-accepted regional techniques, in obstetrics they have several disadvantages. The combined spinal-epidural anaesthesia technique can reduce or eliminate some of the disadvantages of both the epidural technique (e.g. unpredictable block, delayed onset, possible toxic reactions) and the subarachnoid technique (e.g. unpredictable level and profound block, hypotension, postdural puncture headache (PDPH)), while preserving their advantages (e.g. fast onset of a reliable block with the flexibility of an epidural catheter to extend the block if necessary in the case of prolonged surgery or inadequate spinal anaesthesia or to provide pain relief in obstetrics and in the postoperative period).[19] The technique uses the appropriate Tuohy needle, which is inserted in the epidural space using the loss-of-resistance to air technique; any fluid that comes back can only be CSF (although many practitioners prefer to use LOR (loss of resistance) saline and distinguish between saline and CSF). A long fine (27-gauge) spinal needle is introduced through the Tuohy needle and advanced until the tip of the spinal needle is felt to penetrate the dura. After correct placement of the spinal needle is confirmed by return of a free flow of CSF, the appropriate dose of local anaesthetic is injected and the spinal needle is then withdrawn. Spinal needle displacement is possible, unless the newer special combined spinal epidural (CSE) kits in which the hub of the spinal needle locks into the hub of the Tuohy needle are used. After withdrawing the spinal needle, a catheter is introduced about 3–4 cm into the epidural space through the Tuohy needle. Aspiration for blood and CSF is performed, although testing of the exact position of the epidural catheter is very difficult. Even more than with the use of the intermittent technique, careful observation and monitoring of the parturient, while administering small doses of local anaesthetic solution, are necessary.

Catheter penetration through the dural hole is not impossible, but due to recent adjustments ("back eye") not likely. Another recent modification to the optimal length of the spinal needle beyond the tip of the Tuohy needle further improved the technique.

Although the earliest reference to the combined technique appeared in 1937,[20] Brownridge described this technique for use in caesarean deliveries in 1981,[21] and Rawal was the first in 1986 to describe the sequential CSE technique for caesarean deliveries.[22] In this two-stage technique the epidural catheter is not just a reserve catheter, but is actively used to gradually raise the level of an intentional low spinal block. This modification allowed spinal dose titration and reduced the severity and frequency of maternal hypotension.

Other alternatives

Alternatives to epidural anaesthesia for obstetric pain relief during labour and vaginal delivery are, for example, "prepared childbirth", hypnosis, acupuncture, TENS, parenteral opioids, paracervical block, pudendal block, caudal block and inhalational analgesia (50% nitrous oxide in oxygen). These techniques were all very popular during a particular period, although pain relief is achieved far better using epidural analgesia.

In obstetrics, the subarachnoid space may be safely entered, especially nowadays with the availability of pencil-point needles, with a low PDPH rate. Although spinal anaesthesia can be used in vaginal deliveries (e.g. for use in a parturient with severe pain in advanced and very rapidly progressing labour), caesarean deliveries, forceps delivery and postpartum removal of a retained placenta are more often done under subarachnoid anaesthesia. Continuous spinal anaesthesia is another alternative.

The continuous spinal anaesthesia technique can also be used in vaginal deliveries for vaginal delivery, forceps applications, caesarean delivery (if a catheter is already in place), placental extraction and postdelivery episiotomy and/or laceration repairs, but reports on caudal equina syndrome have made anaesthetists more reluctant to use this technique.

Effects of epidural anaesthesia on the progress of labour, motor blockade and instrumental delivery rate

Literature on the effect of epidural anaesthesia reveals that in spontaneous labour, epidural anaesthesia will slightly prolong the first and second stages in both the primiparous and multiparous patient. However, dilute concentrations of local anaesthetics in combination with opioids does not prolong the first or second stage of labour. There is however an increase in instrumental deliveries, due to motor impairment of the abdominal and perineal muscles. Again the use of diluted local anaesthetic solutions has diminished the impact on muscle function, resulting in less malrotations and less instrumental deliveries. The prolongation of the second stage of labour for about 30 minutes does not present any problem in a well monitored labour. However, increased levels of circulating catecholamines (anxiety, fear) are also associated with altered patterns of labour, diminished uterine contractions, decreased uteroplacental perfusion and, possibly, a detrimental effect on the fetus. A discoordinated labour in a parturient with pain is often rapidly altered to a progressive coordinated labour once epidural analgesia is initiated, since epidural block will decrease the level of maternal catecholamines. There is also a wide variation in the obstetric and anaesthetic management of women with epidural anaesthesia, which may explain the wide variations in operative delivery rates in the literature. Variations include the patient populations (e.g. primiparous or multiparous women), the stage at which the epidural is initiated, the choice of the local anaesthetic solution, the concentration and amounts of drugs used, the length of the second stage, whether or not the obstetricians want their patients to feel the distention of their perineal structures so they will "push" better with their contractions in the second stage of labor. Anaesthetists feel that pain relief can be tailored to the needs of the patient and should not be withdrawn from the parturient when she needs it most. Lumbar epidural anaesthesia allows the parturient to cooperate fully with her attendants during labour and delivery and allows her to enjoy more fully the outcome of her efforts. Prolonged pushing could also produce a risk to the fetus.

Anaesthetists often regard motor blockade with epidural labour analgesia as inevitable or of no consequence, although it decreases the parturient's satisfaction. Pain relief has little or no purpose other than patient satisfaction. Modern techniques can result in epidurals which produce pain relief without motor block and with little or no hypotension, a possible reduction in the rate of instrumental vaginal deliveries and long term backache. All these side-effects and associations are related to the amount of bupivacaine given in the form of a test dose, top-ups and infusions throughout labour. Epidural analgesia can range from a barely perceptible sensory block to a block of most of the sympathetic, sensory and motor fibres. The goal of obstetric epidural analgesia is to achieve pain relief without dense sensory block or numbness and loss of motor power. This can only be done by reducing the rate of bupivacaine in milligrams per hour. By injection of the initial analgesic dose into the subarachnoid space by using a combined spinal epidural technique, even if this first dose only consists of opioids alone, the bupivacaine dose throughout labour is diminished considerably compared with a technique where the epidural space only is used. The combination of bupivacaine and opioids also has a synergic effect. Careful guidance of the parturient, giving tailored analgesia, will also result in a diminished use of local anaesthetic. Ambulation is possible, even with a working epidural. The dangers of ambulation with epidural analgesia are possible falls due to motor weakness, hypotension, giddiness or loss of proprioception. Queen Charlotte's Hospital in London has performed more than 5000 mobile epidurals, consisting of a subarachnoid dose of 2·5 mg of bupivacaine with 25 μg fentanyl and maintenance with a 10 ml bolus of 0·1% bupivacaine with 2 μg/ml fentanyl; while no falls were reported all mothers were accompanied by an adult. Anything that eliminates or postpones motor block, increases the woman's sense of being in control during labour with a working epidural. This improves her experience of childbirth without pain.

Side-effects

Vena cava compression syndrome and hypotension

Hypotension is the commonest complication that follows the injection of local anaesthetic into the epidural space. Although several factors may contribute to a decrease in arterial pressure, such as inferior vena caval occlusion (seen in most women in later pregnancy), haemorrhage or vasovagal fainting, the initial trigger to hypotension is the sympathetic blockade caused by the epidural anaesthetic. If the cardiac sympathetics are affected, bradycardia and a reduction in myocardial inotropy will be the result. Acute intravascular volume expansion of the circulation with intravenous fluids should be given together with small doses (5 mg) of ephedrine as vasodilatation is the therapy to treat the primary cause of hypotension. The Kennedy device was specially developed to push away the pregnant uterus in order to avoid the vena cava compression syndrome.[23][24]

Vomiting and nausea

Vomiting and nausea are unpleasant visceral sensations, which often occur in an obstetric patient as a result of elevated levels of progesterone and/or gonadotropins. Mechanical obstruction of the duodenum and upward and backward displacement of the pylorus by the gravid uterus raise the intragastric pressure, render the lower oesophageal sphincter incompetent, delay gastric emptying, increase gastric residual volume, decrease gastric pH and predispose the parturient to gastroesophageal reflux, regurgitation and emetic symptoms. Sympathetic innervation to the stomach (T6–10) may be blocked with high segmental levels of subarachnoid or epidural anaesthesia, leaving relatively unopposed vagal afferent impulses to predominate in the upper gastrointestinal tract. Harsh peritoneal traction, uterine exteriorisation, lower uterine segment stretching or repair by inexperienced surgeons further trigger the vomiting centre. Hypotension and the resultant hypoxaemia of the brain stem vomiting centre may also trigger vomiting. Supplemental oxygen therapy significantly decreases the incidence of emetic symptoms, despite the presence of hypotension. Hypotension should be avoided at all times and aggressively treated if necessary by left-uterine displacement to avoid aortocaval compression, acute hydration and intravenous ephedrine if necessary. Opioid administration to a labouring woman further delays gastric emptying time to twice that of the non-pregnant woman, stimulates the chemoreceptor trigger zone and sensitises the vestibular apparatus to the effects of motion. Intravenous naloxone can reverse the opioid-induced delay of gastric emptying in parturients given opioids.

Symptoms of heartburn and reflux of gastric acids are common during pregnancy. Pregnant women, and especially those women who have heartburn or received opioids, have a weaker lower oesophageal sphincter tone. Antiemetics, such as metoclopramide, domperidone and cyclizine, are known to increase the lower oesophageal sphincter tone, and are also potent dopamine antagonists. They also act at the chemoreceptor trigger zone, which is richly innervated with dopaminergic receptors, and is situated on the floor of the fourth ventricle in the medulla in close proximity to the vomiting centre. Psychogenic and emotional disturbances or unpleasant stimuli may also trigger the vomiting centre. A reassuring compassionate anaesthetist may significantly decrease the incidence of anxiety and related emetic symptoms in a well-informed patient. The administration of metoclopramide, which has antiemetic properties, increases the lower oesophageal sphincter tone and reverses gastric stasis, and this should be considered when a parturient describes a prior history of emesis, symptoms of motion sickness or when opioids are used.[25]

Peripartum emetic symptoms are multifactorial in nature. A management scheme to successfully reduce the incidence of emetic symptoms must anticipate those stimuli or events that may provoke or trigger this response. Metoclopramide is a useful antiemetic whether given before or after caesarean delivery, as a result of its central antidopaminergic activity on the chemoreceptor trigger zone.[26 27] Maternal and fetal safety has been well documented with metoclopramide.[28 29] Adverse side-effects to metoclopramide are dose related and occur infrequently in the 10- to 20-mg dose ranges used clinically.[26 30]

The ideal antiemetic drug for the parturient undergoing caesarean delivery under regional anaesthesia, probably does not exist. If antiemetics are used, proper timing is important. Metoclopramide 10 mg given intravenously, 5–10 minutes before atropine administration, may counter its undesirable effects on the lower oesophageal sphincter tone.[31]

The recently introduced serotonin antagonists (5-HT$_3$-receptor antagonists), ondansetron, tropisetron and granisetron, seem to be more powerful antiemetics than the currently used antiemetics, but their use in pregnant patients is still questionable, because of a lack of studies.

Pruritus

Opioids have excitatory effects, facilitating hyperalgesia and itch. Pruritus, associated with the administration of opioids, is often localised in the face, but can affect the whole body. It is a sensation that provokes the desire to scratch and can be aroused by a variety of mechanical, electrical and chemical stimuli. If patients do experience pruritus with regional anaesthesia, it is often helpful to decrease the demand dose or lock-out interval, change from one opioid to another, or give antihistamines as hydroxyzine or diphenhydramine. Naloxone, naltrexone, nalbuphine and butorphanol have also been used with varying efficacy to decrease the occurrence of pruritus and nausea.

Urinary retention

Increased residual volume and urinary retention are known side-effects of regional anaesthesia. The effect of regional anaesthesia on the post-partum bladder is controversial. Epidural anaesthesia may delay normal voiding, by suppressing afferent sensory impulses from the bladder and inhibiting the reflex mechanism for micturition. Even a single episode of overdistention of the bladder may produce urethrovesicular dysfunction due to irreversible damage to the detrusor muscle. Among contributory factors in reducing bladder problems are avoiding active labour and obstetric traumata and the use of a urinary catheter in order to avoid bladder distention. Although specific studies on urinary retention following epidural/spinal opioids are lacking in obstetrics, a prevalence of urinary dysfunction following epidural morphine has been reported. Possible explanations may be that morphine travels rostrally in the CSF to the supraspinal structures at the level of the pons, where it causes an inhibitory effect on the primary micturition centre; a spinal site of action through autonomic inhibition of sacral parasympathetic outflow; or, the presence of opioid receptors in the urinary bladder which cause a direct effect on bladder relaxation. Treatment includes the opioid antagonist naloxone, or the synthetic cholinergic agonist, betanecol. Frequent checks to determine bladder distention following epidural and subarachnoid anaesthesia are necessary, while catheterisation is indicated in the post-caesarean delivery period or if spontaneous voiding is unsuccessful.

Backache

Backache is a common complaint after parturition, although it is no more common following an epidural anaesthetic, but the insertion of a large needle in the back establishes a strong link in the mother's mind. Backache is a symptom, not a disease, it has many aetiologies, and is frequently treated with epidural injections.

In a recent editorial in the *BMJ*, Russell and Reynolds stated that women should be reassured that no prospective study on the use of regional analgesia in labour has been associated with an increased risk of chronic backache.[32]

Complications

Toxicity of local anaesthetics

An unintentional intravascular injection of local anaesthetic (with toxic reaction) is possible in the gravid parturient near term, in whom the epidural veins are markedly dilated making entry even more likely. Accidental rapid intravenous injection of a large amount of local anaesthetic will result in a grand mal convulsion and possibly cardiovascular collapse. To complicate matters further, epidural catheters that have been functioning normally at a previous injection may migrate into epidural veins or into the subarachnoid space.

The CNS and cerebrovascular system are particularly sensitive to the toxic effects of local anaesthetics. At non-toxic blood levels, minimal CNS effects are observed, but as the dose and subsequent blood levels increase, signs and symptoms may be seen. Mild CNS effects include lightheadedness, dizziness, tinnitus, disorientation and drowsiness. Slurred speech, shivering, muscle twitching and tremors of the face and extremities appear to be the immediate precursors of a generalised convulsive state. If the blood levels of local anaesthetics still increase, CNS excitation will be followed by depression, including respiratory depression and arrest. The potential CNS toxicity of local anaesthetics following an unintentional intravenous injection is correlated with their intrinsic anaesthetic potency (e.g. procaine is the least potent and least toxic of the clinically useful local anaesthetics, while bupivacaine and tetracaine are the most potent compounds). Other factors, such as rate of absorption, tissue distribution and metabolism, also influence toxicity. The more potent local anaesthetics also have a proportional ability to depress cardiac contractility (e.g. bupivacaine, tetracaine and etidocaine depress ventricular contractility by 25% at concentrations of ± 1–$1\cdot 5$ mg/ml, while lidocaine, mepivacaine and prilocaine require concentrations of ± 10–15 mg/ml to cause a similar decrease of 25% in the maximum rate of tension development). The ratio of the dosage required for irreversible cardiovascular collapse and the dosage that will produce CNS toxicity (convulsions), i.e. CC/CNS ratio, is lower for bupivacaine and etidocaine than for lidocaine. Ventricular arrhythmias and fatal ventricular fibrillation may occur following the rapid intravenous administration of a larger dose of bupivacaine but not lidocaine. The pregnant woman may be more sensitive to the cardiotoxic effects of bupivacaine than the non-pregnant patient. Cardiac resuscitation is more difficult following bupivacaine-induced cardiovascular collapse, and acidosis and hypoxia markedly potentiate the cardiotoxicity of bupivacaine.

Cardiac arrest in the parturient

Cardiac arrest in late pregnancy or during delivery is a rare event. Some of its causes in the parturient at term are: total spinal block; local anaesthetic toxicity from unintentional intravascular injection; trauma; pulmonary embolism; and amniotic fluid embolism.

The resuscitation of a pregnant patient at term is unlikely to be successful unless vena cava compression is eliminated. Cardiopulmonary resuscitation (CPR) of the parturient in a "wedged position" should begin with securing the airway. If aggressive CPR with a properly positioned patient is not successful after a short interval, immediate caesarean delivery must be performed as soon as possible. This procedure will immediately relieve the vena caval obstruction from the gravid uterus and increase the chance of survival for both the infant and the mother. CPR (even open chest cardiac compressions) must be continued throughout the procedure until spontaneous and effective cardiac activity occurs, for example, it may take more than 1 hour of cardiac resuscitation in the case of bupivacaine toxicity. Controlled ventilation may have to be continued an even longer period of time.

High epidural block

An epidural block ascending to the upper thoracic and lower cervical segments (producing a Claude–Bernard–Horner syndrome) can be seen with epidural block. If respiratory paralysis occurs, artificial ventilation may be necessary.

Dural puncture

The perforation of the dura mater by an epidural Tuohy needle may produce a tear rather than a puncture hole, depending on the sharpness of the needle used. A clear gush of CSF is usually seen coming out of the needle hub. This should not be confused with physiological saline, if the loss of resistance to saline is used to locate the epidural space. PDPH is very likely the result in obstetric patients. If this is not recognised after inserting the needle, the puncture may become manifest after the catheter has been inserted through the needle. Fluid running back through the catheter will provide the diagnosis, although the catheter end must be lowered below the point of insertion to allow the CSF to escape by gravity. A further diagnostic aid is the use of a test dose. If the catheter tip is within the subarachnoid space, a small dose of local anaesthetic will rapidly produce evidence of developing spinal anaesthesia. Because a test dose containing adrenaline is also used to diagnose intravenous placement of the catheter, a sufficient dose has to be injected; for example, 3–5 ml of 2% lidocaine or 2–3 ml of 0·5% bupivacaine with adrenaline. Sufficient time should be allowed (4–5 minutes) for a spinal block to develop. Evaluation should be for numbness (sensory anaesthesia) and not motor paralysis. Complications of dural puncture are PDPH and the production of high or total spinal anaesthesia. It is estimated that between 20 and 30% of dural punctures are not detected at the time they are done. Equally 20–30% of obvious dural taps do not cause headaches.

An unintentional subdural or subarachnoid injection of local anaesthetic is at best an embarrassment and at worse a life-threatening complication, which if not recognised immediately requires prolonged resuscitation. If a substantial dose of local anaesthetic drug (epidural analgesia requires 8–10 times the dose used for spinal anaesthesia) is injected into the subarachnoid space, a (very) high block will be produced with hypotension, bradycardia, inadequate respiration, or apnoea and unconsciousness. Management consists of ventilation with oxygen, intubation, and increasing arterial pressure and heart rate with an intravenous vasopressor (e.g. ephedrine or adrenaline).

Therefore, some of the *recommended safety procedures* against unintentional subarachnoid or intravenous injection, include:

- Have resuscitation equipment and drugs at hand and an intravenous infusion in place before instituting the anaesthetic
- Monitor the patient adequately, including maternal heart rate and blood pressure, and uterine contractions
- Insert the Tuohy needle using the midline technique and aspirate for blood or CSF before and after placing the catheter (remove bacterial

JET LIBRARY

filter)

- Lower the epidural catheter below the operating table, as gravity may help blood to enter the epidural catheter when a vein is penetrated
- Check the epidural drug yourself, colour code any connection site and identify tubing in order to prevent unintentional addition of medication into the epidural line
- Use a pharmacological test dose containing sufficient local anaesthetic plus adrenaline and wait for several minutes while carefully observing and talking to the patient to detect subjective signs and symptoms
- Give only fractionated doses, inject slowly and allow sufficient time to elapse between the incremental doses.

There is no substitute for close observation of the patient by someone who is trained to detect adverse effects. The anaesthetist should always be highly suspicious that, in spite of a negative result, misplacement can still be present.

Complications from the use of opioids

Perispinal administration of opioids is a powerful and simple technique to potentiate local anaesthetic effects, improving pain relief in obstetrics. However its use is associated with a small but definite risk of respiratory depression, which can occur at unpredictable times. The incidence of respiratory depression, pruritus, urinary retention, nausea and vomiting can be reduced by infusions of low concentrations of naloxone (5 μg/kg/h) or nalbuphine. When large doses of intraspinal morphine are used, monitoring is absolutely necessary. The use of more lipid-soluble opioids (fentanyl-sufentanil-alfentanil) appears to be much safer. In obstetrics, "mini-doses" of opioids are effective and safe and produce (in combination with local anaesthetics) excellent pain relief for long periods of time. Parturients should be monitored with appropriate nurses who are aware of the side-effects associated with pain relief. Apnoea monitors and pulse oximetry are practical and essential if appropriate nursing personnel are not available.

Late complications of epidural anaesthesia

Postdural puncture headache

PDPH usually occurs after an inadvertent dural puncture by a Tuohy needle. The headache is related to a low CSF pressure, especially when the patient sits up or stands. The brain becomes less well supported within the cranium and traction is exerted on the structures supporting it. The condition is related to the amount of CSF leakage from the spinal subarachnoid space to the epidural space, from where it is easily absorbed. The size and shape of the hole caused by the epidural needle puncture is of significant importance. PDPH is likely to be greater than 50%, due to the hole produced by a 16- or 18-gauge Tuohy needle. PDPH can be very severe and incapacitating, accompanied by neck pain and stiffness, leaving the mother unable to enjoy her new baby. An epidural blood patch, injecting 10–20 ml of autologous blood, is by far the most rapid and effective treatment, with a success rate of over 90%. The introduction of new spinal needles for subarachnoid anaesthesia (e.g. pencil point needles) has significantly decreased the incidence of PDPH following subarachnoid anaesthesia.

Neurological complications

Trauma of a single spinal nerve by the needle or catheter, causing disruption of nerve fibres, can occur. The subsequent neuritis can last for some weeks or months. The patient usually complains of pain during insertion of the needle or catheter and at the start of the injection. After the block has worn off, the patient complains of paraesthesia in the distribution of the nerve concerned, with possibly a partial loss of sensation and some motor weakness.

Adhesive arachnoiditis, resulting in permanent loss of spinal cord function, usually follows the injection of an irritant solution (e.g. detergent, KCl, $CaCl_2$, thiopental, sodium bisulphite).

Anterior spinal artery syndrome, due to failure of the blood supply in the distribution of the artery, causes an infarct of the spinal cord with resultant permanent paraplegia.

Space-occupying lesions (e.g. haematomas, abscesses, tumours) can press upon the spinal cord and cause serious cord damage. Large and dangerous haematomas, in the absence of a clotting defect, are extremely rare. In most cases of epidural abscesses, the patient is suffering from a pyrexial disease. The injection of contaminated material into the epidural space appears to be amazingly rare. Local anaesthetics themselves are bacteriostatic or bacteriocidal. Spinal tumours can cause paraplegia by direct pressure, and their presence may not be suspected until full neurological recovery fails to occur after epidural block. If persistent painful backache appears or the nerve block does not fully disappear in the expected time, the possibility of a space-occupying lesion should be excluded or demonstrated by MRI. Urgent laminectomy may prevent permanent damage. In any case of neurological damage ask for full neurological examination and follow-up.

Caesarean deliveries

Premedication

Thirty millilitres of 0·3 mol/l sodium citrate administered before the induction of an anaesthetic in vaginal deliveries is optional, but essential in caesarean deliveries, which are also given metaclopramide 10 mg intravenously and cimetidine 200 or 400 mg or ranitidine 50 mg intramuscularly or intravenously in the 30–60 minutes prior to induction, in order to avoid Mendelsohn's syndrome.

Techniques for caesarean deliveries

Caesarean deliveries are one of the most frequent inpatient surgical procedures performed. Besides general anaesthesia, epidural, subarachnoid and the combined spinal-epidural anaesthesia technique are all suitable for caesarean deliveries.

It is well known that regional anaesthesia has many advantages over general anaesthesia. It allows the mother to stay awake and interact with her infant and partner during the surgical procedure, and she can maintain her own airway with less risk of airway complications, for example aspiration or difficulties with intubation. It avoids neonatal depression if the incision-to-delivery interval becomes prolonged. The incidence of venous thrombosis is less in patients receiving regional anaesthesia. General anaesthesia has only a limited role in emergency caesarean deliveries (e.g. in abruptio placentae, ruptured uterus, placenta previa, bleeding, shock). The Report on Confidential Enquiries into Maternal Deaths in England and Wales is a unique medical audit published triennally, which reviews all maternal deaths. This report indicates that anaesthesia remains a common cause of maternal death, and to date over 75% of these deaths have occurred at the time of emergency general anaesthesia for caesarean delivery.[33] Subarachnoid anaesthesia is a good alternative in the following situations: anticipated airway/intubation problems, history of asthma, diagnosis of upper respiratory infection, recent solid food intake and the mother's wish to remain awake. It is also preferable for the obese woman, those with an anatomically difficult back, and even in cases of fetal compromise.

Epidural anaesthesia offers an excellent degree of controllability with predictable levels of anaesthesia, and the use of an epidural catheter can be helpful in adjusting the degree of surgery, anaesthesia, and sympathetic block.

The regional anaesthesia techniques used are the same as those used for vaginal deliveries, except for the doses of the local anaesthetic solution, which need to be adjusted, and monitoring of the patient which should be the same as for other surgical interventions. Examples of the choices of local anaesthetic for epidural use are: lidocaine 2%, bupivacaine 0·5%, ropivacaine 0·75%, and 2-chloroprocaine 3%. The addition of adrenaline and an opioid may help to increase the quality of the block and decrease the onset time of surgical anaesthesia. A pain-free caesarean delivery usually needs a block which includes an upper sensory block to T5 or T4. Subarachnoid anaesthesia for caesarean deliveries can be obtained with the use of lidocaine 2% or bupivacaine 0·5%, to which opiates are added. The combination of both epidural and subarachnoid techniques offers excellent possibilities for the normal and high-risk obstetric patient, who has to undergo a caesarean delivery.

Looking after the baby

At birth, a fetus has to make the complex physiological transition to a neonate successfully. The asphyxial stress of birth is mild to moderate, and usually the neonate is able to compensate for it. When the neonate's compensatory ability is decreased or the asphyxial stress is excessive, resuscitative intervention is necessary to assist in the conversion from fetal to neonatal physiology. Six per cent of at-term newborns require life support and this percentage increases quickly with low birth weight, especially under 1500 g.

Transient hypoxaemia or acidosis is well tolerated by a newborn baby and prompt intervention usually prevents permanent sequelae. Prolonged neonatal hypoxaemia or acidosis impedes the transition from fetal to neonatal physiology. The fetus/neonate initially responds to hypoxaemia by redistributing blood flow to the heart, brain and adrenal glands, while tissue oxygen extraction increases and myocardial contractility and cardiac output decrease. Hypoxaemia and acidosis promote patency of the ductus arteriosus and persistent pulmonary hypertension with little or no ventilatory drive, which requires prompt intervention.

Fetal heart rate monitoring

Ante- and intrapartum fetal assessment will reveal 80% of cases in which neonatal resuscitation will be necessary. As you will never know beforehand what will happen, fetal assessment must continue throughout labour as the clinical situation can change rapidly. *Fetal heart rate (FHR)* monitoring (fetal scalp electrode monitoring) is most reliable in confirming fetal well-being and is more than 90% accurate in predicting a 5-minute Apgar score >7. In predicting fetal compromise, FHR monitoring has a false positive rate of 35–50%. FHR evaluations include baseline heart rate, baseline heart rate variability and identification of heart rate decelerations. Bradycardia, mediated by increased vagal activity, is the first response to acute hypoxaemia. If hypoxaemia is prolonged, catecholamine release may produce fetal tachycardia, which also can be caused by maternal fever, intrauterine infection or maternal administration of β-adrenergic receptor agonists or anticholinergic agents. Repetitive late decelerations are a sign of fetal stress. *Fetal scalp pH determination* can confirm or exclude fetal acidosis. If the FHR on the cardiotocograph suggests the baby is becoming

Table 4.1   Normal-term neonatal blood gas data (± 1 SD). (Reproduced from Yeomans ER, Hauth JC, Gilstrap LC III. Umbilical cord pH, P_{CO_2}, and bicarbonate following uncomplicated term vaginal deliveries. *Obstet Gynecol* 1985;**151**:879)

	Umbilical vein	Umbilical artery
P_{O_2} (mmHg)	29·2±5·9	18·0±6·2
P_{CO_2} (mmHg)	38·2±5·6	49·2±8·4
pH	7·35±0·05	7·28±0·05
Bicarbonate (mmol/l)	20·4±2·1	22·3±2·5

hypoxic, then a normal pH and P_{O_2} will provide reassurance that the fetus is still compensating for the stress of labour and labour can be allowed to continue. The fetal pH is considered normal if >7·25; pH values between 7·20 and 7·25 indicate a state of preacidosis and <7·20 indicates acidosis. In determining fetal condition, the popularity of the fetal scalp pH technique has declined since the development and the widespread use of cardiotocographic instruments.

In our hospital a fetal scalp pH >7·25 is considered good. If it is less, other factors are taken into consideration before performing a caesarean section: what is the cervical dilatation, how is the fetus, how is the cardiotocograph, how long is the woman *in partu*, . . .? Therefore it is not just a simple question and state that a caesarean delivery should be done below a certain pH or P_{O_2}. This would simplify the problem too much.

Of course the information derived from cardiotocography and fetal blood sampling and pH measurement must always be taken in the context of other labour events, and normal values cannot in any way be regarded as a guarantee of fetal well-being. Situations in which cardiotocography should be recommended include prolonged, induced or augmented labours; multiple pregnancies; thick meconium staining of the amniotic fluid; labour with a known or suspected growth-retarded or preterm fetus; abnormalities of the FHR detected on auscultation; and where epidural anaesthesia is being used. *Pulse oximeter saturation readings* obtained after birth, taken from the baby, provide a good index of neonatal cerebral oxygenation.

Intrapartum resuscitation

Intrapartum resuscitation should be performed once fetal compromise is identified. Maternal factors that impair oxygen delivery to the fetus must be corrected, including maternal aortocaval compression, hypotension, sympathectomy, haemorrhage or cardiac disease. Hyperstimulation, tetany and abruption or rupture of the uterus will also interfere with blood flow to the fetus. Stop oxytocin infusion and administer a tocolytic agent, which will reduce uterine tone and, if abruption or rupture are severe, rapid delivery will be required. Umbilical cord prolapse or compression (e.g. in case of oligohydramnios) and thick meconium may be alleviated by saline amnioinfusion.

Optimisation of fetal oxygenation

Oxygen is of paramount importance for the fetus in order to survive. The fetal Pao_2 is only one-third or one-fourth the maternal Pao_2. Increasing the latter will raise both the umbilical vein and artery Pao_2 levels. Acute loss of O_2-carrying capacity leads rapidly to fetal distress. Blood transfusion therefore is necessary if the haematocrit falls below 28%. Cigarette smoking results in carboxyhaemoglobinaemia, which can be detected in both the mother and fetus. This results in less available haemoglobin for oxygen, a leftward shift of the O_2 dissociation curve, and nicotine-induced utero-placental vasoconstriction. Cessation of smoking at least 48 hours prior to delivery is of paramount importance.

Excessive hyperventilation is hazardous for both the mother and the fetus. The augmentation in maternal respiratory rate may be seen in response to pain, fear and anxiety. The resultant maternal respiratory alkalosis may cause cerebral and uteroplacental vasoconstriction with decreased blood flow, leading to syncope and maternal oxygen debt. The O_2 dissociation curve shifts to the left and impairs the release of O_2 to maternal tissues and fetal blood (up to 23% fall in fetal arterial Pao_2, an increase in fetal base deficit, lower 1-minute Apgar scores, and a delay in sustained respirations). Pain relief (e.g. epidural analgesia) will abolish this excessive hyperventilation; also maternal hypo- and aventilation lead to fetal hypoxaemia. Therefore continuous monitoring of fetal assessment is necessary before delivery and maternal hyperoxia should be maintained until the reason for its use has been eliminated. Fewer newborns require resuscitation and have better 1-minute Apgar scores when 100% oxygen is delivered to the mother. Also under epidural or subarachnoid anaesthesia, it is essential to administer oxygen to the mother, resulting in a beneficial outcome for the fetus (greater fetal O_2 contents and lower base deficit). The greater fetal O_2 content acts as a reservoir which permits the neonate to withstand postnatal apnoea or O_2 deprivation during suctioning of the airway.

Oxygen administration during general anaesthesia for caesarean delivery should never be lower than 50% (preferably 65–100%), even in low risk patients. In fetal distress or in high risk parturients, a FIo_2 of $1·0$ is recommended. The same regimen should be applied during regional anaesthesia. A 6 litre/min flow by mask with reservoir bag will supply a FIo_2 of $±0·50$, a 10 litre/min flow will supply a FIo_2 of $±0·99$, provided a normal ventilatory pattern is assumed, avoiding hyperventilation. As there is no O_2 transmission to the fetus after uterine incision, maternal hyperoxia is indicated until delivery of the baby. Maternal hyperoxia increases the oxygen gradient across the placenta, with an increased O_2 transfer to the fetus, which is beneficial in all circumstances.

Neonatal resuscitation

At birth, neonatal resuscitation includes minimising heat loss, assessment of neonatal respiration, and heart rate. Cold stress leads to hypoxaemia, hypercarbia and metabolic acidosis. The newborn should be dried immediately, using a radiant warmer, and the mouth and nose suctioned briefly (20 seconds). Start positive-pressure ventilation (40–60 breaths/min with 100% oxygen) if the baby is gasping or apnoeic. The laryngeal mask airway size 1 has been used successfully to resuscitate newborns. The majority of neonates requiring any resuscitation will respond to these first steps. Neonatal cardiac arrest is generally secondary to respiratory failure producing hypoxaemia and tissue acidosis, with bradycardia, decreased cardiac contractility and arrest as a result. Severely asphyxiated newborns, who need chest compression, occur in less than 1 in 1000 births. Chest compressions, using the thumb method or the two-finger method, combined with adequate ventilation, normalise cardiac function quickly in almost any situation. New guidelines recommend 90 compressions per minute (instead of 120), at a 3:1 ratio of compressions to ventilations. Although the Apgar score has been used for many years and is still used for prognostic purposes, it is not very helpful in the practical approach to resuscitation. Resuscitation should start immediately if necessary and one should not wait for the 1-minute Apgar score to begin resuscitation. If the heart rate remains below 80 beats/min, despite adequate ventilation and chest compressions, medications are indicated (e.g. naloxone in case of maternal opioid administration, sodium bicarbonate if metabolic acidosis is present despite adequate ventilation, adrenaline to stimulate the heart in an hypotensive, acidotic and bradycardic infant). Adrenaline is the drug of choice if the heart rate is below 80 beats/min despite adequate ventilation and chest compression (intravenous or intratracheal dose: 0·01–0·03 mg/kg or 0·1–0·3 ml/kg of a 1:10 000 solution). Medication can be administered through a peripheral vein, endotracheal instillation or the umbilical vein (insert the catheter until the tip is just below the skin level). Some 10% of healthy term neonates have transient hypoglycaemia (also seen in diabetic mothers, or in mothers who received large amounts of intravenous dextrose) and should be given dextrose 2 g/kg intravenous push, followed by 5–8 mg/kg/min.

Summary

Understanding neonatal physiology and the transition from fetal to neonatal life, pre- and intrapartum fetal assessment of risk factors and intra- and postpartum resuscitation, are of vital importance for the well-being of any neonate.

Regional anaesthesia has an excellent safety record in obstetrics. Epidural anaesthesia is undoubtedly the most effective technique in producing adequate pain relief during vaginal childbirth. The development of newer spinal needles has helped to avoid PDPH, so that subarachnoid anaesthesia is nowadays very popular for caesarean deliveries. In summary, the combination of the epidural and subarachnoid techniques has proved to be advantageous both during labour and delivery.

References

1 Morrison LMM, Wildsmith JAW, Ostheimer GW. In: Van Zundert A, Ostheimer GW, eds, A history of pain relief in childbirth. In: *Pain relief and anesthesia in obstetrics*. Edinburgh: Churchill Livingstone, 1966:3–16.

2 Jouppila R, Jouppila P, Hollmén A, Kuikka J. Effect of segmental extradural analgesia on placental blood flow during normal labour. *Br J Anaesth* 1978;50:563–6.

3 Aburel E. La topographie et le méchanisme des douleurs de l'accouchement avant la période de l'expulsion. *CR Soc Biol (Paris)* 1930;103:902.

4 Cleland JGP. Paravertebral anesthesia in obstetrics. Experimental and clinical basis. *Surg Gynecol Obstet* 1933;57:51–62.

5 Bonica JJ. Peripheral mechanisms and pathways of parturition pain. *Br J Anaesth* 1979;51:3S.

6 Bonica JJ. The nature of pain in parturition. In: Van Zundert A, Ostheimer GW, eds, *Pain relief and anesthesia in obstetrics*. Edinburgh: Churchill Livingstone, 1996;19–52.

7 Lefèbre L, Carli G. Parturition pain in non-human primates: pain and auditory concealment. *Pain* 1985;21:315.

8 Lundh W. Modraundervisning, Forlossningstraining eller foraldrakunskap? PhD dissertation, Pedagogiska Institutionenen, Stockholm Universitet, 1974.

9 Melzack R. The myth of painless childbirth. *Pain* 1984;19:321.

10 Shnider SM. Adverse effects of labour pain on the fetus. In: Van Zundert A, Ostheimer GW, eds, *Pain relief and anesthesia in obstetrics*. Edinburgh: Churchill Livingstone, 1996;53–60.

11 Van Zundert AAJ. Bupivacaine 0·125% plus epinephrine 1:800 000. The value of a low concentration of a local anesthetic drug for epidural analgesia in obstetrics. PhD Thesis, Leiden, The Netherlands, 1985.

12 Van Zundert A, Vaes L, Soetens M. Which syringe for epidurals? *Acta Anaesthesiol Scand* 1988;32:353–4.

13 Van Zundert A, Vaes L, Soetens M, De Wolf A. Identification of inadvertent placement of an epidural catheter in obstetric anesthesia. *Anesthesiology* 1988;68:142–5.

14 Van Zundert A, Vaes L, De Wolf A. ECG monitoring of mother and fetus during epidural anesthesia. *Anesthesiology* 1987;66:584–5.

15 Van Zunder A, Vaes L, Soetens M, *et al.* Every dose given in epidural analgesia for vaginal delivery can be a test dose. *Anesthesiology* 1987;67:436–40.

16 Van Zundert A, Burm A, Van Kleef J, *et al.* Plasma concentrations of epidural bupivacaine in mother and newborn: 0·125% versus 0·375%. *Anesth Analg* 1987;66:435–41.

17 Vertommen J, Vandermeulen E, Van Aken H, *et al.* The effects of the addition of sufentanil to 0·125% bupivacaine on the quality of analgesia during labor and on the incidence of instrumental deliveries. *Anesthesiology* 1991;74:809–14.

18 Van Zundert A, van der Aa P, Van der Donck A, Meeuwis H, Vaes L. Motor blockade, expulsion times and instrumental deliveries with epidural analgesia for vaginal delivery. *Obstet Anesth Digest* 1984;4:152–6.

19 Rawal N, Van Zundert A, Holmström B, Crowhurst JA. The combined spinal–epidural technique. *Reg Anaesth* 1997;22: (Sept/Oct issue).

20 Soresi AL. Episubdural anesthesia. *Anesth Analg* 1937;16:306–10.

21 Brownridge P. Epidural and subdural analgesia for elective cesarean section. *Anaesthesia*

1981;**36**:70.

22 Rawal N. Single segment combined spinal epidural block for cesarean section. *Can J Anaesth Soc J* 1986;**33**:254–5.

23 Kennedy RL. An instrument to relieve inferior vena cava occlusion. *Am J Obstet Gynecol* 1970;**107**:331–3.

24 Colon-Morales MA. A self-supporting device for continuous left uterine displacement during cesarean section. *Anesth Analg* 1970;**49**:223–4.

25 Lussos SA, Johnson MO. Peripartum nausea and emesis. In: Van Zundert A, Ostheimer GW, eds, *Pain relief and anaesthetics in obstetrics*. Edinburgh: Churchill Livingstone, 1996;249–56.

26 Lussos SA, Bader AM, Thornhill M, Datta S. The antiemetic efficacy of prophylactic metoclopramide for cesarean delivery. *Soc Obstet Anesth Perinatol*, Abstracts, 1991.

27 Chestnut DH, Vandewalker GE, Owen CL. Administration of metoclopramide for prevention of nausea and vomiting during epidural anesthesia for elective cesarean section. *Anesthesiology* 1987;**66**:563.

28 Frame WT, Allison RH, Moir DD, Nimmo WS. Effect of naloxone on gastric emptying during labour. *Br J Anaesth* 1994;**56**:263.

29 Bylsma-Howell M, Riggs KW, McMorland GH. Placental transport of metoclopramide: assessment of maternal and neonatal effects. *Can Anesth Soc J* 1983;**30**:487.

30 Tornetta FJ. Clinical studies with the new antiemetic, metoclopramide *Anesth Analg* 1969;**48**:198.

31 Brock-Utne JG, Rubin J, Downing JW. The administration of metoclopramide with atropine. *Anaesthesia* 1976;**31**:1186.

32 Russell R, Reynolds F. Back pain, pregnancy and childbirth. *BMJ* 1997;**314**:1062–3.

33 to be completed at proof stage.

Selected reading

Ostheimer GW. *Manual of obstetric anesthesia*, 3rd edn. Edinburgh: Churchill Livingstone, 1994.

Shnider SM, Levinson G. *Anesthesia for obstetrics*, 3rd edn. Baltimore: Williams and Wilkins, 1991.

Van Zundert A, Ostheimer GW. *Pain relief and anesthesia in obstetrics*. Edinburgh: Churchill Livingstone, 1996.

5: Management of acute paediatric pain

ISABELLE MURAT

The undertreatment of paediatric pain has been recognised for nearly 10 years.[1-4] Indeed after either major or minor surgery, children were receiving much less doses of narcotics than adults for similar painful procedures.[5] Since that time, many editorials, reviews and textbooks have focused on pain therapy in infants and children,[6-10] but receipts are not always easy to use on a daily basis. This is true, even in adults, as demonstrated by a large survey conducted on a one-day basis in April 1994 in all adult surgical wards in Paris (unpublished data). This survey demonstrated that post-operative pain was still described as severe by 46% of patients, especially after major surgical procedures such as spinal, upper abdominal, or renal surgery. After the initial prescription of analgesics performed by the anaesthetists in the recovery room, very few orders were changed afterwards. In paediatric patients, similar results can be expected. The difficulties are even worse in children owing to the poor verbal language in infants and young children together with fears of respiratory depression, fears of addiction in older children, the lack of parental presence, as well as the environmental conditions of the recovery room (noise, contention, residual effect of anaesthetic agents . . .).[11]

Evaluation of postoperative pain in children

Pain perception may be modified by many situational, emotional and behavioural factors (Fig. 5.1).[12] Difficulty in evaluation of pain is one of the most important reasons for undertreatment of paediatric postoperative pain.[13-17] In children over 5 years of age, self-assessment using the simple numerical rating score, the VAS, the Oucher scale, the poker chip tools or the Faces scale, is the most reliable. All these methods have some drawbacks. The youngest children often have difficulty relating their pain on a VAS, especially after surgery, and the concept of a VAS is often too abstract.[18] The faces represented on both the Faces scale and on the Oucher scale may be interpreted as representing pain as well as other emotional

119

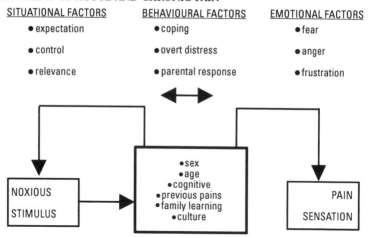

SITUATIONAL FACTORS
- expectation
- control
- relevance

BEHAVIOURAL FACTORS
- coping
- overt distress
- parental response

EMOTIONAL FACTORS
- fear
- anger
- frustration

NOXIOUS STIMULUS

- sex
- age
- cognitive
- previous pains
- family learning
- culture

PAIN SENSATION

Fig 5.1   A model of the situational, behavioural and emotional factors that modify a child's pain perception[12]

factors such as parental separation or an unfriendly environment.[19] For preverbal children, behavioural observation scales have been evaluated. The oldest one is the CHEOPS (Children's Hospital of Eastern Ontario Pain Scale) (Table 5.1) designed to evaluate postoperative pain in children 1–5 years of age.[20] The Objective Pain-Discomfort Scale (OPDS) (Table 5.2) measures both physiological and behavioural responses to pain.[21 22] Both scoring systems are useful to evaluate the efficacy of pain treatments in young children, but less useful on a daily basis. Indeed, differentiation between anxiety and pain may be very difficult to assess. The Observer Pain Scale (Table 5.3) is the most common scale used by nurses in the recovery room. Despite their relative simplicity, all these scales are underused in the postoperative period, except for research purpose.

Analgesic agents and techniques in paediatrics

Peripheral analgesics

Paracetamol (acetaminophen) and NSAIDs are commonly used after standard surgical procedures in children. These agents are however not strong enough for major procedures. Acetyl salicylic acid is no longer used for postoperative pain treatment owing to its adverse effects on the gastrointestinal tract and platelet function, as well as its possible implication in the aetiology of Reye syndrome.

Paracetamol (acetaminophen)

Paracetamol (acetaminophen) is used primarily as an antipyretic drug in children. Its analgesic effect is both peripherally and centrally medi-

120

Table 5.1   Condensed version of the Children's Hospital of Eastern Ontario Pain Scale (CHEOPS) for postoperative pain in children 1–5 years of age

Item	Behavioural definition	Score
Cry	No cry	1
	Moaning, whimpering	2
	Full-lunged cry, sobbing	3
Facial expression	Smiling, definite positive facial expression	0
	Neutral facial expression	1
	Grimace, definite negative facial expression	2
Verbal expression	Child talks about other things, no complaints	0
	Child does not speak	1
	Child complains about pain	2
Torso motility	Body at rest	1
	Body in motion, shaking, arched, or rigid	2
	Body in upright position	3
Wound touching	Child does not attempt to touch wound	1
	Child attempts to touch wound	2
Leg motility	Relaxed leg position or gentle movements	1
	Restless, kicking movements	2
	Standing, crouching, or kneeling	2

ated. It is devoid of unwanted side-effects on haemostasis as well as on renal and gastrointestinal functions. Liver toxicity is only observed after massive overdose, and is less likely to occur in children compared with adults.[23][24] In the postoperative period, paracetamol can be given orally, rectally, or

Table 5.2   Objective pain-discomfort scale (OPDS)

Item	Criteria	Score
Blood pressure (systolic)	±10% preoperatively	0
	>10–20% preoperatively	1
	>20% preoperatively	2
Crying	Not crying	0
	Crying but responds to tender loving care (TLC)	1
	Crying and does not respond to TLC	2
Movement	None	0
	Restless	1
	Thrashing	2
Agitation	Asleep or calm	0
	Mild	1
	Hysterical	2
Verbal evaluation or body language (preverbal child)	Asleep or states no pain	0
	No special posture	0
	Mild pain or cannot localise	1
	Flexing extremities	1
	Moderate pain and can localise, holding location of pain	2

Table 5.3 The Observer Pain Scale (OPS)

Item	Score
Laughing, euphoric	1
Happy, contented	2
Calm or asleep	3
Mild to moderate pain:	
crying, grimacing, restlessness; can distract with toy, food, parental presence	4
crying, screaming, inconsolable	5

intravenously. The intravenous preparation, propacetamol, is a pro-drug which is rapidly hydrolysed to paracetamol, such that 1 g propacetamol produces 0·5 g of paracetamol.[25] It should be given over 15 minutes to be the most effective. The plasma concentrations of paracetamol associated with antipyretic effect have been determined but those required to produce analgesia have not been evaluated. The optimal dosage of paracetamol for postoperative analgesia remains to be determined. The dosage recommended by the International Association for the Study of Pain (IASP) is 20 mg/kg of paracetamol given rectally every 4 hours or 15 mg/kg orally every 4–6 hours (Table 5.4). These dosages seem to be insufficient according to recent paediatric clinical studies.[26–28] After administration of a single rectal dose of 40 mg/kg, maximal concentration was achieved at $2·3 \pm 1·3$ h (mean $\pm$ SD), and plasma levels were above antipyretic values for 6 hours.[26] Similar data were obtained after 35 mg/kg rectal paracetamol,[27] whereas insufficient plasma concentrations were obtained after 10 and 20 mg/kg rectal paracetamol.[28] These data suggest that after an initial rectal dose of 35–40 mg/kg of paracetamol, the subsequent doses (20–30 mg/kg) should be given every 6 hours. For the intravenous route, an initial dose of 30 mg/kg of propacetamol provides effective plasma concentrations for 4 hours. No accumulation was observed for 24 hours in children, in whom the elimination half-life is shorter than in adults (mean values ranging between 1·6 and 2 hours).[25]

Non-steroidal anti-inflammatory drugs (NSAIDs)

NSAIDs are increasingly used for postoperative pain management in children and in adults since the introduction of ketorolac. The latter is no longer available in some European countries (France, Germany), as the incidence of its adverse effects was found to be unacceptably high, especially in the elderly. Indeed, ketorolac as well as all NSAIDs may promote gastrointestinal dysfunction (pain and bleeding), may increase postoperative bleeding, and may favour the occurrence of renal insufficiency. For these reasons, their use should be restricted to the early postoperative period, and they should be used with caution in patients with pre-existing renal or gastric disorders as well as after haemorrhagic surgery.

Table 5.4 Guide to dose of analgesics in paediatric patients[124]

Drug	Route of administration	Dose	Author's comments
Paracetamol	Oral	10–15 mg/kg q 4 h	30 mg/kg q 6 h? (see text)
	Rectal	15–20 mg/kg q 4 h	
Propacetamol	IV	30 mg/kg q 6 h	1 g propacetamol = 0·5 g paracetamol
Aspirin	Oral	10–15 mg/kg q 4 h	Effects on platelets and GI tract
Ibuprofen	Oral	3–10 mg/kg q 6 h	NSAIDs adverse effects
Codeine	Oral	0·5–1 mg/kg q 4 h	The IM route is no longer recommended
			Should be prescribed with paracetamol
Morphine	Oral	0·2–0·4 mg/kg q 4–6 h	
	Oral slow release	0·3–0·6 mg/kg q 12 h	
	IV bolus	0·02–0·1 mg/kg q 2 h	The IM route is no longer recommended
	PCA bolus	0·015 mg/kg q 8 min	
	IV infusion	0·01–0·02 mg/kg/h	Neonates
	IV infusion	0·01–0·06 mg/kg/h	Child
Pethidine	IV	0·2–1 mg/kg q 2 h	The IM route is no longer recommended
	IV infusion	0·2 mg/kg/h	Neonates (accumulation of Norpethidine
			may produce seizures)
	IV infusion	0·2–0·6 mg/kg/h	Child
Fentanyl	IV	0·5–1·5 µg/kg q 0·5 h	
	IV infusion	1–2 µg/kg/h	
Nalbuphine	IV	0·2 mg/kg q 4–6 h	
	IV infusion	0·05 mg/kg/h	

GI = gastrointestinal; IM = intramuscular; IV = intravenous; PCA = patient-controlled analgesia.

NSAIDs are especially effective after orthopaedic or maxillofacial surgery and following all surgical procedures involving large tissue trauma.[29-31] Their use after ENT surgery has been challenged by the potential risk of postoperative bleeding.[32-36] Suppositories of diclofenac were found to be better than paracetamol alone for analgesia following adenoidectomy without an increase in postoperative bleeding.[34] However, in this particular study the dose of paracetamol used was insufficient (10 mg/kg rectally). In another investigation comparing ketorolac (1 mg/kg intravenously) and rectal paracetamol (35 mg/kg) given preoperatively,[33] the authors found no differences in postoperative pain scores and postoperative analgesic requirements, whereas the use of NSAIDs was associated with an increase in peroperative bleeding. Diclofenac was less effective than papaveretum following tonsillectomy, and postoperative bleeding was increased.[35] Ketorolac (1 mg/kg) was compared with morphine (0·1 mg/kg) to provide postoperative pain relief in children after tonsillectomy.[36] Ketorolac reduced the number of emetic episodes after postanaesthesia care unit (PACU) discharge, but increased the likelihood of major bleeding in the first 24 hours after surgery. All these studies suggest that the use of NSAIDs may increase bleeding during and/or after haemorrhagic surgery.

The opioid sparing effects of NSAIDs has been evaluated only after minor surgery in children.[37] Although the use of postoperative narcotics was decreased in the early postoperative period in children receiving NSAIDs during surgery, this study should be repeated after major surgery before definite conclusions can be drawn.

Opioids

Morphine remains the first-line drug after major surgery in children, whereas other opioids may be useful for common surgical procedures.

Agonist-antagonists

Nalbuphine is an antagonist of μ-receptors and an agonist of κ-, σ- and δ-receptors. Nalbuphine is widely used in infants and children for postoperative analgesia.[38] Nalbuphine is thought to be safer than pure μ-agonist agents, as it has lesser respiratory depressant effects than morphine. The ceiling effect explains why nalbuphine is less effective than morphine for major surgery, and why respiratory depression is most of the time not detected in clinical practice. However, as for all other opioids, respiratory depression may occur when nalbuphine is combined with sedative drugs or tranquillisers. Nalbuphine can be administered either intermittently (0·2 mg/kg q 4–6 h) or by continuous infusion after a loading dose (0·2 mg/kg followed by 1 mg/kg/day). Nalbuphine may be given rectally (0·3 mg/kg q 4–6 h) when intravenous access no longer exists. This route of administration is of particular value in emergency services. Owing to its antagonist activity on μ-receptors, nalbuphine may be used to reverse some adverse effects of opioids (urinary retention, pruritus) without modifying their efficacy on pain relief.[39][40] In this particular indication, lower doses of nalbuphine are employed (0·1 mg/kg intravenous bolus or 0·5 mg/kg/day intravenous infusion).

Weak opioids (WHO level 2 agents)

Weak opioids represent an alternative to agonist-antagonists, especially because oral preparations are available. The availability of such drugs may differ from one country to another. Codeine is one of the most popular drugs. Commercial preparations of a combination of paracetamol and codeine are now available. Papaveretum is popular in the UK but unavailable in other European countries. Tramadol seems to be a promising agent. Its affinity for opioid μ-receptors is 10 times lower than that of morphine, and most of its analgesic effect seems to be due to non-opioid effects. Indeed, experimental and clinical data suggest that tramadol may also exert its analgesic effect through direct modulation of monoaminergic pathways. As a consequence, it has less respiratory depressant effects than morphine at equianalgesic doses, and clinical experience has confirmed so far that tramadol is an effective and relatively safe analgesic that may be of value in several pain conditions not requiring treatment with strong opioids.[41][42]

Intravenous morphine

Intravenous morphine remains the first-line treatment of pain after major surgery.[8] Morphine is administered either intermittently, by continuous infusion, or using PCA pumps. The intramuscular route is no longer recommended. The subcutaneous route may be an alternative to intravenous administration when an intravenous access no longer exists.[43] The plasma concentrations of morphine required to attain analgesia or adequate sedation during long term infusion in patients in paediatric intensive care units (PICU) appear to be dependent on the age of the patient. After thoracic or extensive orthopaedic surgery, the mean concentration of morphine necessary to provide an analgesic response was 26 μg/l in infants compared with 4 μg/l in children 2–6 years of age.[44] These data indicate that neonates may be less sensitive to the analgesic effect of morphine than older children (see below). Other investigators have reported effective analgesic plasma concentrations to be 12 μg/l for postoperative analgesia and 65 μg/l for intraoperative analgesia in children. At the same morphine plasma concentration, no age-related differences in respiratory effects were observed in patients aged 2–570 days.[45] Continuous infusion of morphine has been used for analgesia in the intensive care unit for a number of years, as patients are closely monitored for complications and the sedative effects of morphine facilitate controlled ventilation. However, morphine infusion may be used in spontaneously breathing children. After cardiac surgery,

Lynn et al[45] demonstrated that continuous infusions of morphine at 10–30 µg/kg/h provided satisfactory analgesia and did not interfere with spontaneous ventilation, even though there was a five-fold variation in measured morphine serum levels. Continuous morphine infusion is very effective after major surgery in infants and children. Owing to the development of PCA techniques, continuous infusion is usually reserved for children who are not able to run PCA pumps.

Extensive clinical experience with morphine infusions has shown that provided patients are adequately observed, respiratory depression is very uncommon.[43-47] Careful attention to the degree of sedation is vital (see below).[48] The respiratory depressant effect of morphine is however less important at equianalgesic doses than that of pethidine or buprenorphine.[49 50]

Patient-controlled analgesia (PCA)

PCA is the best means of providing pain relief after major surgery.[51 52] This mode of administration allows individual titration of intravenous morphine according to pain intensity. Morphine consumption depends on the surgical procedure, and on individual pain perception. There is a considerable variability between patients as well for each individual patient during the postoperative course.[48 53] The key point for running PCA devices in children is to select the patients appropriately. In order to use PCA effectively, a child must:

1 Have an ability to push the button
2 Understand the relationship between pushing the button and medication delivery
3 Trust that the amount of medication being delivered is in a safe range
4 Understand that expected outcome is pain control, not elimination of pain.[8]

In some particular conditions, children as young as 4–5 years of age are able to correctly use a PCA pump, but most of the patients should be aged over 8 years to fully benefit from the technique. The method should be explained to both children and parents during the preoperative visit. The latter should be instructed not to press the button, which has to be activated only by the child. Morphine is the drug of choice for PCA. Morphine should first be titrated in the recovery room. After an initial bolus of 0·1 mg/kg, an additional bolus of 0·025 mg/kg is given every 5 minutes until satisfactory pain relief is achieved. Standard orders are as follows: 4 hour limit 0·4 mg/kg, bolus 0·015–0·020 mg/kg, refractory period 6–8 minutes. Bolus-only administration often results in disappointing pain relief and sedation. Background infusion (5–15 µg/kg/h) is not recommended in adults, but it is very useful in children.[54-57] The latter reinforces the credibility of the system, and the child is no longer alone for managing its pain. Standard orders should be re-evaluated twice daily according to pain intensity, the number of valid demands, and the incidence and the severity of adverse effects. Three parameters have to be monitored: pain, sedation, and respiratory frequency.[48] Oximetry is required for major upper abdominal or thoracic surgery. Pain is evaluated usually with the VAS. The level of sedation is important to consider, as excessive sedation is the earliest sign of overdose. Respiratory frequency is said to be a poor indicator of respiratory depression. This parameter is however especially important when children are asleep during night. The warning thresholds vary according to the age: 15 bpm in children under 5 years of age, 10 bpm in children over 6. A written protocol for naloxone administration should be available at the bedside. It should be indicated on the order chart that no sedatives or tranquillisers should be given without calling the doctor in charge of the patient.

The other adverse effects are those of opioids. Nausea and vomiting are common during the first 24 hours,[58] and may be decreased by metoclopramide, droperidol or nalbuphine. Prophylactic hyoscine patches are very effective in reducing the incidence of opioid-related nausea and vomiting at the expense of a dry mouth and some increase in sedation. Intestinal paralysis is always observed and should be treated after 48 hours. Urinary retention is observed in 30–50% of patients. If a bladder catheter was inserted for surgery, it should be maintained for the first 24 hours. Otherwise, naloxone or nalbuphine should be titrated at the bedside until urinary retention has resumed.

Nurse control analgesia may be used in young children. The nurses are asked to provide the bolus to the child according to pain intensity. This is a costly method compared with standard intravenous infusion pumps. *Mother control analgesia* is useful for handicapped children, as mothers are more likely to understand pain manifestations than nurses or doctors facing the child for the first time.

Spinal opioids

Opioids may be administered epidurally alone or with local anaesthetics, or on rare occasions intrathecally. Even when administered via the caudal route, preservative-free epidural morphine has been shown to provide effective and prolonged postoperative analgesia following abdominal, thoracic and cardiac surgery in children.[59–62] The risk of delayed respiratory depression related to the rostral spread of epidural morphine[63] should be minimised by selecting the minimum effective dose. In most published studies, not a single case of respiratory depression was observed. The incidence of other opioid-related undesired side-effects is however very high, ranging from 25 to 50% for nausea and vomiting and from 15 to 50% for urinary retention.[64] All the published cases of respiratory depression have been observed when doses of morphine greater than 0·05 mg/kg were used.[65][66] The administration of 0·033, 0·067 or 0·1 mg/kg of morphine sulphate by the caudal route produced analgesia lasting 10, 10·4 and 13·3 hours respectively, and the incidence of side-effects was similar in the three groups.[61] As the duration of analgesia increases only marginally with increasing the dose of epidural morphine, administration of the smallest effective dose should be considered. This minimum effective dose seems to be close to 0·03 mg/kg.[67] The risk of respiratory depression seems to be greater in infants of less than 12 months of age than in older children. Valley and Bailey[65] have reported 11 cases of respiratory depression in 138 administrations of caudal morphine (0·07 mg/kg). All were observed within 12 hours (mean 3·8 hours) of morphine administration, and 10 were in children 12 months of age or younger. However most of those infants had received intravenous narcotics intraoperatively for major surgery. Despite the limitation of this study, this suggests that infants of less than 12 months of age should be fully monitored in the PICU when epidural opioid treatment is considered. Other more lipophilic opioids, such as fentanyl or sufentanil, are mostly used in combination with local anaesthetics (see below).

Intrathecal administration of morphine has been proposed in selected patients, particularly after cardiac surgery or spinal surgery.[68–72] After 0·025 mg/kg intrathecal morphine, analgesia lasted 36–72 hours following spinal surgery, but at the expense of some degree of respiratory depression in most patients. Lower doses of 0·007–0·035 mg/kg seem to be as effective at reducing the risk of delayed respiratory depression. Nevertheless, this technique should be reserved for selected patients monitored for 48 hours in a critical care setting.

Other routes of administration

New routes of administration have been proposed for opioid administration—the transmucosal and the transdermal routes.

Fentanyl is now available for transmucosal administration (Oralet®).[73][74] This preparation has been mainly evaluated as premedication. From the few studies available so far, it seems that a dose of transmucosal fentanyl of 10–15 μg/kg given preoperatively provides similar postoperative analgesia for tonsillectomy as 2 μg/kg of intravenous fentanyl given during surgery.[75] Further studies are required to determine the place and the safety of this new preparation for postoperative pain relief in children.

Transdermal patches of fentanyl have been proposed for postoperative pain treatment. Absorption is slow, and maximal plasma concentration is not achieved before several hours. After patch removal, plasma concentration decreases slowly. Therefore, the clinical effect and the occurrence of side-effects may be delayed and long lasting. In addition, each patch contains a definite dose of fentanyl, which does not allow for precise weight-basis prescription. Fentanyl patches delivering 25 μg/h have been used after cardiac surgery in children aged 18–60 months.[76] In this particular study, maximal plasma concentration was achieved 18 hours after placement of the patch. Postoperative analgesia was deemed adequate in those patients carefully monitored in the PICU. This mode of administration seems more interesting for managing chronic pain than for postoperative pain treatment.

Special concerns in the neonate

Neonates seem to be less sensitive to the analgesic effects of opioids than infants, children and adults, whereas they are more sensitive to their respiratory depressant effects.[77] This phenomenon is thought to be related to both pharmacokinetic and pharmacodynamic developmental differences.[78] It has been suggested that respiratory depression and analgesia produced by μ-agonists involve different receptors subtypes.[79] These receptors change in number in an age-related fashion. Indeed, 14-day-old rats are 40 times more sensitive to morphine analgesia than 2-day-old rats, but morphine depresses the respiratory rate in 2-day-old rats to a greater degree than in 14-day-old rats.[80] Although these data may not be true in humans, there is clinical evidence that the newborn are particularly sensitive to the respiratory depressant effects of the commonly administered opioids. The pharmacokinetics of opioids varies greatly during infancy (Table 5.5).[44 81–85] Total body clearance of all opioids is low in preterm infants and neonates and increases during the first year of life. For example, morphine clearance increases from values ranging between 0·5 and 3 ml/kg/min in preterm infants to values ranging between 20 and 40 mg/kg/min in preschool children.[44] The increased permeability of the blood–brain barrier in the neonatal period explains why cerebral concentrations of morphine are greater in neonates than in older children.[86 87] For all these reasons, neonates, and particularly preterm neonates, may be susceptible to the effects of morphine, which emphasises the importance of individual dosage titration.[88] As a result, use of any narcotics in the

Table 5.5 Clearance values (ml/kg/min) of some opioids according to age[44]

Age	Morphine	Pethidine	Fentanyl	Alfentanil	Sufentanil
1–7 days					
Preterm	2·7–9·6	3·5	12·1	0·9–2·9	—
Term	2·3–20·0	7·2	9–28	1·7	4·2
1 week–2 months	7·4–9·0	9·7	22·4	—	6·7–17
2–12 months	11·4–33·5	—	18·1–30·6	8·2–11·5	21·5–27·5
1–6 years	6·2–56·2	10·4	11·5–12·8	4·7–11·1	16·9–30·5
7 years	6·7–25·7	—	7·1	8·2	12·8–16·4
Adults	12–34	10–12	12–15	5·4–8·3	12·7

newborn calls for close monitoring and supervision of the patient after administration of the drug.

Regional anaesthesia

Regional techniques are increasingly used for providing intra- and postoperative analgesia for minor and major surgery in children. Single shot techniques are employed for minor procedures whereas major surgery requires catheter placement.

Single shot techniques

Single shot techniques are routinely used for minor surgery, often performed on outpatients.[89] Both central blocks and peripheral blocks are used. Caudal anaesthesia is the most popular block in infants and children.[90] Indications are all the surgical procedures below the umbilicus lasting less than 90 minutes. When caudal block is performed before surgery, opioid administration is unnecessary, thus reducing the incidence of postoperative nausea and vomiting. Caudal anaesthesia provides excellent postoperative analgesia for 4–6 hours after surgery. The duration of postoperative analgesia is identical whether the caudal block is performed before surgery or at the end of surgery.[91] Analgesia is prolonged when local anaesthetics with adrenaline are used instead of plain solutions. The addition of adrenaline is more effective in increasing the duration of postoperative analgesia in young children than in older children.[92] The duration of intra- and postoperative analgesia is markedly prolonged by the addition of clonidine to local anaesthetics (see below). Caudal anaesthesia does not delay voiding after surgery.[93] For minor surgical procedures, prolonged motor blockade and urinary retention have to be avoided in the postoperative period. Therefore solutions with a low concentration of local anaesthetics (0·175–0·25% bupivacaine, 1% mepivacaine or 1% lidocaine) are strongly recommended.

Other simple regional techniques have been proved to be very useful for providing pain relief after surgery. Ilioinguinal block is as effective as caudal anaesthesia for pain relief after hernia repair.[94–96] It is an alternative to caudal block when the latter is contraindicated or has failed. Local wound infiltration is another alternative to regional techniques for providing postoperative pain relief after minor surgery (hernia repair, appendicectomy).[94 97 98] Penile block is mainly used for circumcision.[99 100] Although it is very effective, postoperative analgesia lasts only several hours and additional analgesics are required for the first 24 hours after surgery.[101] Femoral block is indicated for fractured femoral shaft. It may be performed in an emergency to allow for pain-free X-ray examination and transportation.[102] Axillary block is indicated for hand surgery. Even a single shot provides long lasting analgesia.

Catheter techniques

Catheters are required for long lasting surgical procedures to permit additional injection of local anaesthetics and/or for painful surgical procedures such as some orthopaedic surgical procedures in which early physiotherapy is mandatory. Caudal catheters should be removed at the end of surgery owing to their high risk of septic contamination in the postoperative period. Trans-sacral, lumbar or thoracic catheters can be left in place for providing postoperative analgesia.[103] In the postoperative period, analgesia can be provided either by intermittent top-up injections or by continuous infusion using 0·125% or 0·1% bupivacaine. The latter is theoretically a better choice as it avoids the recurrence of pain. The risk of toxicity during continuous infusion should be kept in mind, especially in infants. Indeed, toxicity is related to the accumulation of local anaesthetics that will produce high plasma levels of local anaesthetics.[104] The recent report of several life-threatening complications related to the systemic toxicity of local anaesthetics (seizures, myocardial depression)[105 106] has led to the proposal of the following recommendations with regard to local anaesthetic dosing for postoperative continuous infusions:[107]

1 Children are probably not more "resistant" to local anaesthetic toxicity than adults. Indeed the plasma concentrations measured in children with seizures ranged between 2 and 10 μg/ml.

2 Premonitory symptoms of systemic toxicity are often lacking, and restlessness or agitation due to minor CNS toxicity may be misinterpreted in young infants.

3 The extremity of the epidural catheter should be placed in the correct position to reduce the amount of local anaesthetics needed to achieve pain relief. For example, the catheter should be advanced to the thoracic level to provide adequate analgesia after thoracic or upper abdominal surgery.

4 After a loading dose of 2–2·5 mg/kg of bupivacaine (1·5 mg/kg in neonates), infusion rates should not exceed 0·4–0·5 mg/kg/h in children and 0·2–0·25 mg/kg/h in neonates and infants. Bupivacaine 0·1% or 0·125% provides excellent postoperative pain relief with a reduced incidence of motor blockade.

5 The infusion rate should be reduced in children with risk factors for seizures.

6 When analgesia is not sufficient using recommended dosages, the position of the catheter should be checked. If the catheter is correctly placed, opioids should be added to local anaesthetics, whereas the infusion rate of local anaesthetics should not be increased. Conversely, if analgesia is effective, the infusion rate should be decreased after 12 hours of continuous infusion.

Interpleural catheters have been used to provide analgesia after thoracotomy.[108–110] This technique is not always effective, and may lead to excessive plasma levels of local anaesthetics.

Adjuvants to local anaesthetics

The addition of adrenaline to local anaesthetics increases the duration of analgesia after single shot techniques, especially when long lasting local anaesthetics such as bupivacaine are used. This effect is more important in young children than in older children. The use of adrenaline-containing solutions is not recommended for continuous infusion techniques. Opioids are often combined with local anaesthetics to improve postoperative analgesia. The addition of morphine to local anaesthetics is very effective,[111 112] whereas the addition of fentanyl to local anaesthetics remains controversial.[113–116] The addition of fentanyl does not affect markedly the duration of postoperative analgesia,[116] but it allows the use of low concentrations of bupivacaine (0·625% to 0·1%), thus reducing the risk of unwanted motor blockade. The risk of opioid-related adverse effects should always be considered even if lipophilic opioids such as fentanyl or sufentanil are used.[117]

The addition of clonidine, an α2-agonist, to local anaesthetic increases markedly the duration of postoperative analgesia. The time to additional analgesia is nearly doubled when clonidine is added to standard doses of bupivacaine.[118 119] For inguinal hernia repair, the addition of clonidine (1 µg/kg) to plain bupivacaine increased the duration of postoperative analgesia of more than 8 hours in children aged 1–7 years.[118] After orthopaedic surgery, postoperative analgesia lasted 12 hours in children receiving bupivacaine plus clonidine (2 µg/kg), whereas additional analgesics were required after 4 hours in those receiving plain bupivacaine.[119] No adverse effects commonly observed in adults (hypotension) were obvious in children. As the respiratory depressant effects of clonidine are minimal,[120] the addition of clonidine seems to be a very effective and safe technique to increase the duration of local anaesthetic-related analgesia.

Strategy for postoperative pain therapy

Planning postoperative pain treatment is basically a part of anaesthetic management. Therapeutic options will mainly depend on the age of the child, on the surgical procedure involved, on the postoperative monitoring facilities available, and finally on the analgesic technique used during surgery (opioids or regional anaesthesia). Several therapeutic options may be used for a given child and a given procedure, and the risk/benefit ratio of the technique and/or of the agent chosen should always be considered.

The majority of minor surgical procedures are carried out on outpatients. The children should not be sent home without a written order for supplementary analgesics. Both paracetamol and NSAIDs are easy to administer, either by the oral or rectal route. The quality of postoperative analgesia can be assessed by questioning the parents about the quality of sleep during the first postoperative night. Minor procedures such as circumcision or cryptorchidy may be extremely painful after regional block has worn off.[101]

For major surgery, the choice among the different techniques of analgesia mainly depends on the monitoring facilities available. The use of PCA pumps does not require special monitoring facilities. Most of the children are safely monitored in standard wards, and do not require continuous pulse oximetry monitoring. Children having thoracic or upper abdominal surgery are often monitored in the PICU, in which monitoring facilities as well as trained nursing staff are available. Continuous epidural infusion may be used in normal surgical wards provided that trained nursing staff and reliable syringe pumps are available. Children having major surgery should be evaluated twice daily in order to assess the quality of pain relief as well as the incidence of side-effects of pain treatment.

Dedicated paediatric pain services are very useful for improving the quality of postoperative analgesia and providing pain relief for complex cases.[121 122] They are run by consultant anaesthetists with designated sessions for acute pain relief, and clinical nurse specialists. Nurse specialists are pivotal to the success of an acute pain service, because they motivate ward nurses, develop nursing protocols for specific analgesic techniques, institute ward nurse education, and supervise the development of patient observation. The development of paediatric pain services is a major advance in improving postoperative analgesia.

Finally, surgery is not the only source of pain during the postoperative period. Repetitive blood samples or physiotherapy are often requested after major surgery and may trigger additional pain. The use of EMLA cream will alleviate pain due to venepuncture, whereas it is often easy to anticipate physiotherapy-related pain with PCA. The administration of an equimolar mixture of nitrous oxide and oxygen (Entonox) is another useful tool for alleviating procedures related to pain, such as removal of a chest tube or dressing change.[123] Procedure-related pain should not be neglected, in order to improve the overall quality of postoperative analgesia.

References

1 Mather L, Mackie J. The incidence of postoperative pain in children. *Pain* 1983;15:271–82.
2 Purcell-Jones G, Dormon F, Sumner E. The anaesthetist's perception of neonatal and infant pain. *Pain* 1988; 33:181–7.
3 Schechter NL. The undertreatment of pain in children: an overview. *Ped Clin North Am* 1989;36:781–94.
4 Dilworth NM. Children in pain: an underprivileged group. *J Pediatr Surg* 1988;23:103–4.

5 Schechter NL, Allen DA, Hanson K. Status of pediatric pain control: a comparison of hospital analgesic usage in children and adults. *Pediatrics* 1986;77:11–5.

6 Weinger MB, Koob GF. What constitutes adequate analgesia in animals? In neonates? *Anaesthesiology* 1990;72:767–8.

7 Yaster M. Analgesia and anesthesia in neonates. *J Pediatr* 1987;111:394–5.

8 Goresky GV, Klassen K, Waters JH. Postoperative pain management for children. *Anesth Clin North Am* 1991;9:801–19.

9 Rodgers MC. Do the right thing. Pain relief in infants and children. *N Engl J Med* 1992;326:55–6 [editorial].

10 Schechter NL, Berde CB, Yaster M. *Pain in infants, children, and adolescents.* Baltimore: Williams and Wilkins, 1993:691 pp.

11 Schechter NL, Bernstein BA, Beck A, Hart L, Scherzer L. Individual differences in children's response to pain: role of temperament and parental characteristics. *Pediatrics* 1991;87:171–7.

12 McGrath PA. Pain assessment in children. A practical approach. In: Tyler DC, Krane EJ, eds, *Advances in pain research therapy*, vol 15. New York: Raven, 1990:5–30.

13 Owens ME. Pain in infancy: conceptual and methodological issues. *Pain* 1984;20:213–30.

14 Porter F. Pain assessment in children and infants. In: Schechter NL, Berde CB, Yaster M, eds, *Pain in infants, children, and adolescents.* Baltimore: Williams and Wilkins, 1993:87–96.

15 Maunuksela EL, Olkkola KT, Korpela R. Measurement of pain in children with self-reporting and behavioral assessment. *Clin Pharmacol Ther* 1987;42:137–41.

16 Beyer JE, Wells N. The assessment of pain in children. *Pediatr Clin North Am* 1989;36:837–54.

17 Mathews JR, McGrath PJ, Pigeon H. Assessment and measurement of pain in children. In: Schechter NL, Berde CB, Yaster M, eds, *Pain in infants, children, and adolescents.* Baltimore: Williams and Wilkins, 1993:97–111.

18 Manne SL, Jacobsen PB, Redd WH. Assessment of acute pediatric pain: do child self-report, parent ratings, and nurse ratings measure the same phenomenon? *Pain* 1992;48:45–52.

19 Bieri D, Reeve RA, Champion GD, Addicoat L, Ziegler JB. The faces pain scale for the self-assessment of the severity of pain experienced by children: development, initial validation, and preliminary investigation for ratio scale properties. *Pain* 1990;41:139–50.

20 McGrath PJ, Johnson G, Goodman JT, Schillinger J, Dunn J, Chapman J. The CHEOPS: a behavioral scale to measure postoperative pain in children. In: Fiels HL, Dubner R, Cervero F, eds, *Advances in pain research and therapy.* New York: Raven, 1985:395–402.

21 Broadman LM, Rice LJ, Hannalah RS. Testing the validity of an objective pain scale for infants and children. *Anesthesiology* 1988;69:A770.

22 Norden J, Hannalah R, Getson P, O'Donnell R, Kelliher G, Walker N. Reliability of an objective pain scale in children. *Anesth Analg* 1991;72:S199.

23 Penna A, Buchanan N. Paracetamol poisoning in children and hepatotoxicity. *Br J Clin Pharmacol* 1991;32:143–9.

24 Rumore MM, Blaiklock RG. Influence of age-dependent pharmacokinetics and metabolism on acetaminophen toxicity. *J Pharm Sci* 1992;81:203–7.

25 Granry JC, Rod B, Boccard E, Hermann P, Gendron A, Saint-Maurice C. Pharmacokinetics and antipyretic effects of an injectable pro-drug of paracetamol (propacetamol) in children. *Paediatr Anaesth* 1992;2:291–5.

26 Anderson BJ, Woolard GA, Holford NHG. Pharmacokinetics of rectal paracetamol after major surgery in children. *Paediatr Anaesth* 1995;5:237–42.

27 Houck CS, Sullivan LJ, Wilder RT, Rusy LM, Burrows FA. Pharmacokinetics of a higher dose of rectal acetaminophen in children. *Anesthesiology* 1995;83:A1126.

28 Birmingham PK, Tobin MJ, Fanta KB, Berkelhamer M, Smith FA, Henthorn TK. 24 hour pharmacokinetics of rectal acetaminophen in children: an old drug with new recommendations. *Anesthesiology* 1995;83:A1127.

29 Maunuksela EL, Ryhanen P, Janhunen L. Efficacy of rectal ibuprofen in controlling postoperative pain in children. *Can J Anaesth* 1992;39:226–30.

30 Campbell WI. Analgesic side effects and minor surgery: which analgesic for minor and

day-case surgery? *Br J Anaesth* 1990;**64**:617–20.

31 Maunuksela EL, Olkkola KT, Korpela R. Does prophylactic intravenous infusion of indomethacin improve the management of postoperative pain in children? *Can J Anaesth* 1988;**35**:123–7.

32 Watters CH, Patterson CC, Mathews HML, Campbell W. Diclofenac sodium for posttonsillectomy pain in children. *Anaesthesia* 1988;**43**:641–3.

33 Rusy LM, Houck CS, Sullivan LJ, *et al*. A double-blind evaluation of ketorolac tromethamine versus acetaminophen in pediatric tonsillectomy: analgesia and bleeding. *Anesth Analg* 1995;**80**:226–9.

34 Baer GA, Rorarius MGF, Kolehmainen S, Selin S. The effect of paracetamol or diclofenac administered before operation on postoperative pain and behaviour after adenoidectomy in small children. *Anaesthesia* 1992;**47**:1078–80.

35 Thiagarajan J, Bates S, Hitchcock M, Morgan-Hughes J. Blood loss following tonsillectomy in children. A blind comparison of diclofenac and papaveretum. *Anaesthesia* 1993;**48**:132–5.

36 Gunter JB, Varughese AM, Harrington JF, *et al*. Recovery and complications after tonsillectomy in children: a comparison of ketorolac and morphine. *Anesth Analg* 1995;**81**:1136–41.

37 Kokki H, Hendolin H, Maunuksela EL, Vainio J, Nuutinen L. Ibuprofen in the treatment of postoperative pain in small children. A randomized double-blind placebo controlled parallel group study. *Acta Anaesthesiol Scand* 1994;**38**:467–72.

38 Wandless JG. A comparison of nalbuphine with morphine for post-orchidopexy pain. *Eur J Anaesthesiol* 1987;**4**:127–32.

39 Penning JP, Samson B, Baxter AD. Reversal of epidural-induced respiratory depression and pruritus with nalbuphine. *Can J Anaesth* 1988;**35**:599–604.

40 Cohen SE, Ratner EF, Kreitzman TR, Archer JH, Mignano LR. Nalbuphine is better than naloxone for treatment of side effects after epidural morphine. *Anesth Analg* 1992;**75**:747–52.

41 Vickers MD, O'Flaherty D, Szekely SM, Read M, Yoshizumi J. Tramadol: pain relief by an opioid without depression of respiration. *Anaesthesia* 1992;**47**:291–6.

42 Houmes RJ, Voets MA, Verkaaik A, Erdmann W, Lachmann B. Efficacy and safety of tramadol versus morphine for moderate to severe postoperative pain with special regard to respiratory depression. *Anesth Analg* 1992;**74**:510–4.

43 McNicol R. Postoperative analgesia in children using continuous s.c. morphine. *Br J Anaesth* 1993;**71**:752–6.

44 Olkkola KT, Hamunen K, Maunuksela EL. Clinical pharmacokinetics and pharmaco-dynamics of opioid analgesics in infants and children. *Clin Pharmacokinet* 1995;**28**:385–404.

45 Lynn AM, Nespeca MK, Opheim KE, Slattery JT. Respiratory effects of intravenous morphine infusions in neonates, infants, and children after cardiac surgery. *Anesth Analg* 1993;**77**:695–701.

46 Hendrickson M, Myre L, Johnson DG, Matlak ME, Black RE, Sullivan JJ. Postoperative analgesia in children: a prospective study of intermittent intramuscular injection versus continuous intravenous infusion of morphine. *J Pediatr Surg* 1990;**25**:185–91.

47 Koren G, Butt W, Chinyanga H, Soldin S, Tan YK, Pape K. Postoperative morphine infusion in newborn infants: assessment of disposition characteristics and safety. *J Pediatr* 1985;**107**:963–7.

48 Morton NS. Development of a monitoring protocol for safe use of opioids in children. *Paediatr Anaesth* 1993;**3**:179–84.

49 Hamunen K, Olkkola KT, Maunuksela EL. Comparison of the ventilatory effects of morphine and buprenorphine in children. *Acta Anaesthesiol Scand* 1993;**37**:449–53.

50 Hamunen K. Ventilatory effects of morphine, pethidine and methadone in children. *Br J Anaesth* 1993;**70**:414–8.

51 Rodgers BM, Webb CJ, Stergios D, Newman BM. Patient-controlled analgesia in pediatric surgery. *J Pediatr Surg* 1988;**23**:259–62.

52 Berde CB, Lehn BM, Yee JD, Sethna NF, Russo D. Patient-controlled analgesia in children and adolescents: a randomized, prospective comparison with intramuscular administration of morphine for postoperative analgesia. *J Pediatr* 1991;**118**:460–6.

53 Tyler DC, Pomietto M, Womack W. Variation in opioid use during PCA in adolescents. *Paediatr Anaesth* 1996;6:33–8.

54 Doyle E, Robinson D, Morton NS. Comparison of patient controlled analgesia with and without a background infusion after lower abdominal surgery in children. *Br J Anaesth* 1993;71:670–3.

55 Skues MA, Watson DM, O'Meara M, Goddard JM. Patient-controlled analgesia in children. A comparison of two infusion techniques. *Paediatr Anaesth* 1993;3:223–8.

56 Doyle E, Harper I, Morton NS. Patient controlled analgesia with low dose background infusions after lower abdominal surgery in children. *Br J Anaesth* 1993;71:818–22.

57 Lloyd-Thomas AR. Management of postoperative pain. *Curr Opin Anaesthesiol* 1994;7:262–6.

58 Weinstein MS, Nicolson SC, Schreiner MS. A single dose of morphine sulfate increases the incidence of vomiting after outpatient inguinal surgery in children. *Anaesthesiology* 1994;81:572–7.

59 Jensen BH. Caudal block for postoperative pain relief in children after genital operations. A comparison between bupivacaine and morphine. *Acta Anesthesiol Scand* 1981;25:373–5.

60 Krane EJ, Jacobson LE, Lynn AM, Parrot C, Tyler DC. Caudal morphine for postoperative analgesia in children: a comparison with caudal bupivacaine and intravenous morphine. *Anesth Analg* 1987;66:647–53.

61 Krane EJ, Tyler DC, Jacobson LE. The dose response of caudal morphine in children. *Anesthesiology* 1989;71:48–52.

62 Rosen KR, Rosen DA. Caudal epidural morphine for control of pain following open heart surgery in children. *Anesthesiology* 1989;70:418–21.

63 Attia J, Ecoffey C, Sandouk P, Gross JB, Samii K. Epidural morphine in children: pharmacokinetics and CO_2 sensitivity. *Anesthesiology* 1986;65:590–4.

64 Murat I. Pharmacology. In: Dalens B, ed, *Regional anesthesia in infants, children, and adolescents*. Baltimore: Williams and Wilkins, 1995:67–125.

65 Valley RD, Bailey AG. Caudal morphine for postoperative analgesia in infants and children. A report of 138 cases. *Anesth Analg* 1991;72:120–4.

66 Krane EJ. Delayed respiratory depression in a child after caudal epidural morphine. *Anesth Analg* 1988;67:79–82.

67 Mayhew JF, Bodsky RC, Blakey D, Petersen W. Low-dose caudal morphine for postoperative analgesia in infants and children: a report of 500 cases. *J Clin Anesth* 1995;7:640–2.

68 Jones SEF, Beasley JM, Macfarlane DWR, Davis JM, Hall-Davies G. Intrathecal morphine for postoperative pain relief in children. *Br J Anaesth* 1984;56:137–40.

69 Dalens B, Tanguy A. Intrathecal morphine for spinal fusion in children. *Spine* 1988;13:494–8.

70 Blackman RG, Reynolds J, Shively J. Intrathecal morphine: dosage and efficacy in younger patients for control of postoperative pain following spinal fusion. *Orthopedics* 1991;14:555–7.

71 Harris MM, Kahana MD, Park TS. Intrathecal morphine for postoperative analgesia in children after selective dorsal root rhizotomy. *Neurosurgery* 1991;28:519–22.

72 Nichols DG, Yaster M, Lynn AM, *et al*. Disposition and respiratory effects of intrathecal morphine in children. *Anesthesiology* 1993;79:733–8.

73 Ashburn MA, Lind GH, Gillie MH, de Boer AJF, Pace NL, Stanley TH. Oral transmucosal fentanyl citrate (OFTC) for the treatment of postoperative pain. *Anesth Analg* 1993;76:377–81.

74 Stanley TH, Leiman BC, Rawal N. The effects of oral transmucosal fentanyl citrate premedication on preoperative behavioral responses and gastric volume and acidity in children. *Anesth Analg* 1989;69:328–35.

75 Dsida RM, Wheeler M, Birmingham PK, Fanta KB, Maddalozzo J, Cote CJ. A double blind comparison of the fentanyl Oralet® with IV fentanyl for tonsillectomy. *Anesthesiology* 1995;83:A1180.

76 Paut O, Camboulives J, Tillant D, Levron JC, Viard L. Pharmacokinetics and tolerance of transdermal fentanyl in young children. *Anesthesiology* 1992;77:A1203.

77 Chay PCW, Duffy BJ, Walker JS. Pharmacokinetic–pharmacodynamic relationships of

morphine in neonates. *Clin Pharmacol Ther* 1992;**51**:334–42.

78 Kupfenberg HJ, Way EL. Pharmacologic basis for the increased sensitivity of the newborn rat to morphine. *J Pharmacol Exp Ther* 1963;**141**:105–9.

79 Leslie FM, Tso S, Hurlbut DE. Differential appearance of opiate receptor subtypes in neonatal rat brain. *Life Sci* 1982;**31**:1393–6.

80 Zhang AZ, Pasternak GW. Ontogeny of opioid pharmacology and receptors: high and low affinity site differences. *Eur J Pharmacol* 1981;**73**:29–40.

81 Lynn AM, Slattery JT. Morphine pharmacokinetics in early infancy. *Anesthesiology* 1987;**66**:136–9.

82 McRorie TI, Lynn AM, Nespeca MK, Opheim KE, Slattery JT. The maturation of morphine clearance and metabolism. *Am J Dis Child* 1992;**147**:972–6.

83 Choonara IA, Mckay P, Rane A. Morphine metabolism in children. *Br J Clin Pharmacol* 1989;**28**:599–604.

84 Gauntlett IS, Fisher DM, Hertzka RE, Kuhls E, Spellman MJ, Rudolph C. Pharmaco-kinetics of fentanyl in neonatal humans and lambs: effects of age. *Anesthesiology* 1988;**69**:683–7.

85 Koehntop DE, Rodman RH, Brundage DM, Hegland MG, Buckley JJ. Pharmaco-kinetics of fentanyl in neonates. *Anesth Analg* 1986;**65**:227–32.

86 Lynn AM, McRorie T, Calkins D, Opheim K, Slattery J. Morphine partitioning in a primate model. *Anesthesiology* 1989;**71**:A1067.

87 Way WL, Costley EC, Way EL. Respiratory sensitivity of the newborn infant to meperidine and morphine. *Clin Pharmacol Ther* 1965;**6**:454–61.

88 Gourlay GK, Boas RA. Fatal outcome with use of rectal morphine for postoperative pain control in an infant. *BMJ* 1992;**304**:766–7.

89 Shandling B, Steward DJ. Regional analgesia for postoperative pain in pediatric outpatient surgery. *J Pediatr Surg* 1980;**15**:477–80.

90 Kay B. Caudal block for postoperative pain relief in children. *Anaesthesia* 1974;**29**:610–1.

91 Rice LJ, Pudimat MA, Hannalah RS. Timing of caudal block placement in relation to surgery does not affect duration of postoperative analgesia in paediatric ambulatory patients. *Can J Anaesth* 1990;**37**:429–31.

92 Warner MA, Kunkel SE, Offord KO, Atchinson SR, Dawson B. The effects of age, epinephrine, and operative site on duration of caudal analgesia in pediatric patients. *Anesth Analg* 1987;**66**:995–8.

93 Fisher QA, McComiskey CM, Hill JL, *et al.* Postoperative voiding interval and duration of analgesia following peripheral or caudal nerve blocks in children. *Anesth Analg* 1993;**76**:173–7.

94 Casey WF, Rice LJ, Hannallah RS, Broadman L, Norden JM, Guzzetta P. A comparison between bupivacaine instillation versus ilioinguinal/iliohypogastric nerve block for postoperative analgesia following inguinal herniorrhaphy in children. *Anesthesiology* 1990;**72**:637–9.

95 Hannallah RS, Broadman LM, Belman AB, Abramovitz MD, Epstein BS. Comparison of caudal and ilioinguinal/iliohypogastric nerve blocks for control of post-orchiopexy pain in pediatric ambulatory surgery. *Anesthesiology* 1987;**66**:832–4.

96 Hinkle AJ. Percutaneous inguinal block for the outpatient management of post-herniorrhaphy pain in children. *Anesthesiology* 1987;**67**:411–3.

97 Fell D, Derrington MC, Taylor E, Wandless JG. Paediatric postoperative analgesia. A comparison between caudal block and wound infiltration of local anaesthetic. *Anaesthesia* 1988;**43**:107–10.

98 Wright JE. Controlled trial of wound infiltration with bupivacaine for postoperative pain relief after appendicectomy in children. *Br J Surg* 1993;**80**:110–1.

99 Soliman MG, Tremblay NA. Nerve block of the penis for post-operative pain relief in children. *Anesth Analg* 1978;**57**:495–8.

100 Carlsson P, Svensson J. The duration of pain relief after penile block to boys undergoing circumcision. *Acta Anaesthesiol Scand* 1984;**28**:432–4.

101 Knight JC. Post-operative pain in children after day case surgery. *Pediatr Anaesth* 1994;**4**:45–51.

102 Ronchi L, Rosenbaum D, Athouel A, *et al.* Femoral nerve blockade in children using

bupivacaine. *Anesthesiology* 1989;**70**:622–4.

103 Murat I, Delleur MM, Estève C, Egu JF, Raynaud P, Saint-Maurice C. Continuous extradural anaesthesia in children. Clinical and haemodynamic implications. *Br J Anaesth* 1987;**59**:1441–50.

104 Berde CM. Toxicity of local anaesthetics in infants and children. *J Pediatr* 1993;**122**:S14–20.

105 Agarwal R, Gutlove DP, Lockhart CH. Seizures occurring in pediatric patients receiving continuous infusion of bupivacaine. *Anesth Analg* 1992;**75**:284–6.

106 McCloskey JJ, Haun SE, Deshpande JK. Bupivacaine toxicity secondary to continuous caudal epidural infusion in children. *Anesth Analg* 1992;**75**:287–90.

107 Berde CB. Convulsions associated with pediatric regional anesthesia. *Anesth Analg* 1992;**75**:164–6.

108 McIlvaine WB, Knox RF, Fennessey PV, Goldstein M. Continuous infusion of bupivacaine via intrapleural catheter for analgesia after thoracotomy in children. *Anesthesiology* 1988;**69**:261–4.

109 Tobias JD, Martin LD, Oakes L, Rao B, Wetzel RC. Postoperative analgesia following thoracotomy in children: interpleural catheters. *J Pediatr Surg* 1993;**28**:1466–70.

110 Giaufré E, Bruguerolle B, Rastello C, Coquet M, Lorec AM. New regimen for interpleural block in children. *Paediatr Anaesth* 1995;**5**:125–8.

111 Wolf AR, Hughes D, Hobbs AJ, Prys-Roberts C. Combined morphine-bupivacaine caudals for reconstructive penile surgery in children: systemic absorption of morphine and postoperative analgesia. *Anaesth Intensive Care* 1991;**19**:17–21.

112 Wolf AR, Hughes D, Wade A, Mather SJ, Prys-Roberts C. Postoperative analgesia after paediatric orchidopexy: evaluation of a bupivacaine-morphine mixture. *Br J Anaesth* 1990;**64**:430–5.

113 Lejus C, Roussiere G, Testa S, Ganansia MF, Meignier M, Souron R. Postoperative extradural analgesia in children: comparison of morphine with fentanyl. *Br J Anaesth* 1994;**72**:156–9.

114 Caudle CL, Freid EB, Bailey AG, Valley RD, Lish MC, Azizkhan RG. Epidural fentanyl infusion with patient-controlled epidural analgesia for postoperative analgesia in children. *J Pediatr Surg* 1993;**28**:554–9.

115 Jones RDM, Gunawardene VMS, Yeung CK. A comparison of lignocaine 2% with adrenaline 1:200 000 and lignocaine 2% with adrenaline 1:200 000 plus fentanyl as agents for caudal anaesthesia in children undergoing circumcision. *Anaesth Intensive Care* 1990;**18**:194–9.

116 Campbell F, Yentis SM, Fear D, Bissonnette B. Analgesic efficacy and safety of a caudal bupivacaine–fentanyl mixture in children. *Can J Anaesth* 1992;**39**:661–4.

117 Benlabed M, Ecoffey C, Levron JC, Flaisler B, Gross JB. Analgesia and ventilatory response to CO_2 following epidural sufentanil in children. *Anesthesiology* 1987;**67**:948–51.

118 Jamali S, Monin S, Begon C, Dubousset AM, Ecoffey C. Clonidine in pediatric caudal anesthesia. *Anesth Analg* 1994;**78**:663–6.

119 Lee JJ, Rubin AP. Comparison of a bupivacaine–clonidine mixture with plain bupivacaine for caudal anaesthesia in children. *Br J Anaesth* 1994;**72**:258–62.

120 Penon C, Ecoffey C, Cohen SE. Ventilatory response to carbon dioxide after epidural clonidine injection. *Anesth Analg* 1991;**72**:761–4.

121 Lloyd-Thomas AR. A pain service for children. *Paediatr Anaesth* 1994;**4**:3–15.

122 Shapiro BS, Cohen DE, Covelman KW, Howe CJ, Scott SM. Experience of an interdisciplinary pediatric pain service. *Pediatrics* 1991;**88**:1226–32.

123 Griffin GC, Campbell VD, Jones R. Nitrous oxide–oxygen sedation for minor surgery. Experience in a pediatric setting. *JAMA* 1981;**245**:2411–3.

124 Ready LB, Edwards WT (eds). *Management of acute pain: a practical guide. Task force on acute pain.* Seattle: International Association for the Study of Pain, 1992.

6: Chronic low back pain

RICHARD L. RAUCK

Accurate diagnosis and effective treatment of low back pain represents an enormous medical dilemma for primary care practitioners and specialists. Between 80% and 90% of people are estimated to experience an episode of low back pain at some time in their life.[1 2] A Finnish study estimated the lifetime prevalence of low back pain at 75%.[3] Within this population 50% had experienced an episode of low back pain within the past year and 60% of the population reported some disability attributable to low back pain.

While acute low back pain is considered a self-limiting disease for most individuals, it can progress to total incapacitation and a life of despair for some. Back pain ranks second to upper respiratory tract infections as the most common reason a person seeks medical attention, and is the most common reason a patient visits the orthopaedic surgeon or neurosurgeon.[4 5] Most patients (75–90%) with isolated incidents of low back pain can expect to respond to non-specific treatments within 6 weeks.[6] Recurrence of symptoms approximates 60% of inpatients who experience an episode of low back pain.[7]

The healthcare cost of low back pain is extraordinary. In 1990 the direct costs associated with diagnosing and treating low back pain in the USA were estimated at $23·5 billion.[8] The indirect costs, which included lost working days, added an additional $35 billion to make the total cost approach $60 billion. In a separate study, Nachemson recently estimated that the total cost of low back pain to Sweden in a 1-year period totalled $10 billion.[9]

The high cost of managing chronic low back pain is associated with many treatment failures, and frustrates both patients and practitioners. Many of these failures are attributed to a poor understanding of the aetiology of low back pain. A multitude of structures in the low back can cause pain and it can be extremely difficult to determine which structure acts as the causative agent in a given patient. Similar symptoms can exist for strikingly different pain problems.

The physical examination can often be ambiguous or confounding, and laboratory and radiographic tests do not always correlate with the clinical picture. Determining the exact pain generator which is causing the patient's pain complaint is essential to successful management. This demands a skilled clinician who can take a complete history, perform a thorough physical examination, and accurately interpret laboratory and radiographic findings. Once an accurate diagnosis is made appropriate treatment follows.

Epidemiology

Contrary to inclination the highest age-specific incidence for non-specific, non-mechanical low back pain patients is during the early twenties, and the prevalence continues to increase until the sixth decade of life when a gradual decline begins. It has been postulated that the decline in prevalence during later life represents patients focusing on other health-related problems. Also, morphological changes in the intervertebral disc which occur later in life may make it less susceptible to producing mechanical low back pain symptoms. Non-mechanical causes of low back pain such as osteoporosis and malignancies occur with much greater frequency in the elderly.[4]

In 75–90% of patients with low back pain the natural history results in a resolution of symptoms within 6 weeks with non-specific treatment.[5] It has been estimated that 5% of low back pain patients progress to chronic symptoms, defined simply as pain of greater than 6 months' duration.[6] Why some patients progress to a chronic state remains unclear but is believed to be multifactorial in nature.[10] Whether practitioners can identify non-responders early and afford effective treatment which changes the natural history of chronic low back pain is critical to saving many of the dollars spent on this pain problem. Altering the natural history depends on the ability to recognise and change either the risk factors or prognostic factors[11] (Fig. 6.1).

While it has been believed by many that mechanical factors play a significant role in disability issues, these have not been clearly defined, and specific cause-and-effect relationships have not been demonstrated in any study design.[12] Psychosocial issues play an important role and include job satisfaction, workers' compensation, disability, the chronic illness behaviour role and many others.[13-20]

In a study of 2349 workers' compensation patients with low back pain, 9·7% had a 6-month or longer absence from work.[21] Thirty six per cent of these patients had at least one recurrence of low back pain during a 3-year follow-up period.[22] When further analysed the patients who had an initial episode lasting 3 months or longer had a much greater likelihood of having a prolonged disability during a subsequent low back pain episode.

A comparison of disabling low back pain among countries is presented in Table 6.1.[12 21-24] Recurrence of back pain episodes is common in many of these reports. A back pain episode does not necessarily correlate with lost work, as reported by Biering-Sorensen who found that 70% of subjects reported an episode of low back pain but only 23% stated they had stayed home from work secondary to the pain.[25]

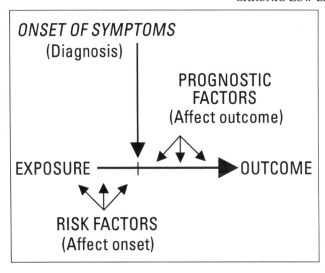

Fig 6.1 Differentiating risk factors from prognostic factors. (Reproduced from Bombadier, *et al.*[11])

Risk factors for low back pain include obesity and occupational factors including lifting and exposure to vibration[26 27] (Table 6.2). Low work satisfaction and boring, monotonous jobs have been associated with higher incidences of back disability in industrial workers.[28] While other social factors such as smoking and lower socioeconomic status have been

Table 6.1 International comparison: yearly incidence of disabling low back pain. (Reproduced from Nachemson[12])

Country	Inhabitants (millions)	Back pain-related days of sickness (million days/yr)	Back diagnoses (% of workforce sicklisted/yr)	Average number of days of back-related absence per patient per year	Level of insurance benefit
USA	240	20	2	9	0–80%
Canada	23	10	2	20	40–90%
Great Britain	55	33	2	30	0–80%
West Germany	61	16	4	10	100% (0–4 weeks) 80% (5–8 weeks) 60% (9 weeks)
The Netherlands	14	4	4	25	80%
Sweden					
1980	8	7	3	25	90%
1983	8	13	5	30	90%
1987	8·5	28	8	40	100%

Figures in parentheses indicate duration of low back pain episode.

Table 6.2   Epidemiological risk factors for onset of work-related low back pain. (Adapted from Bombardier, *et al*[11])

Domain	Risk factors
Demographic factors	Younger age, male sex
Physical work factors	"Heavy" physical work, manual handling (especially lifting), non-neutral trunk postures, whole body vibration
Psychosocial work factors	Low job satisfaction, monotonous work
Medical history	Previous back pain
Physiological	Low fitness level, low trunk strength
Health behaviour	Smoking

associated with higher rates of low back pain, these may not have a cause and effect relationship.[29]

Aetiology/classification

As stated above, the aetiological considerations which produce low back pain symptoms are considered multifactorial. Pathophysiological aspects interplay with the psychosocial aspects in many patients. The severity of an episode, the progression to chronicity, and the disability involve many facets beyond the physical findings.[30–32] The clinician must be able to recognise when these psychosocial factors have become major factors and require referral for psychological intervention.

The practitioner managing low back pain patients must try and determine what physical problem produces the patient's symptoms. Many different structures in the back have the potential to produce pain and these must be separated out in each patient whenever possible. An attempt to answer the question: "What is the pain generator?" should be made for each patient. This requires expert history-taking skills and a thorough physical examination of each patient. The history and physical examination guides the clinician to the appropriate radiographic and laboratory tests.[33–35] Selective, diagnostic nerve blocks can help confirm or refute the diagnosis in some cases.

No classification scheme is perfect for the patient with low back pain[37] (Tables 6.3–6.5). However, one needs to understand the different types of low back pain and how they relate to each other. A broad classification scheme aids in making accurate diagnoses.

Mechanical low back pain

Mechanical low back pain includes a large variety of conditions which produce pain in the low back region.[36 38] This term does not point to a specific diagnosis but does classify the pain symptoms. Tissues believed responsible in the pain of mechanical low back pain are usually relegated to the region of the involved structures, although radiation to buttocks and

142

even the lower extremities can be seen. Patients with mechanical low back pain usually have resolution of their symptoms within 2 weeks, with or without treatment, although a minority (1–5%) will progress to chronic pain syndromes.[39]

Myofascial pain syndromes

Myofascial pain symptoms can develop in muscles throughout the body. These muscles are particularly troublesome in the low back for several reasons. They represent some of the largest muscles in the body and are under significant stress as they maintain a person in the upright posture. They are rather easily subjected to injury from outside mechanical forces, and because of their deep location relative to the skin they can be difficult to treat with local manoeuvres.

Injured muscles of the low back notoriously produce radicular symptoms in some patients[40] (Fig. 6.2). This can easily be confused with sciatica of neuropathic origin. A thorough physical examination and understanding of the referral patterns of myofascial pain syndromes is essential in all patients.

Table 6.3 Classification of low back pain syndromes. (Reproduced from Wheeler[7])

Mechanical or activity-related causes
  Segmental and discal degeneration
  Myofascial or soft tissue injury/disorder
  Disc herniation with possible radiculopathy
  Spinal instability with possible spondylolisthesis or fracture
  Vertebral body fracture
  Spinal canal or lateral recess stenosis
  Arachnoiditis, including postoperative scarring
Systemic disorders
  Primary or metastatic neoplasm, including myeloma
  Osseous, discal or epidural infection
  Inflammatory spondyloarthropathy
  Metabolic bone disease, including osteoporosis
  Vascular disorders such as atherosclerosis or vasculitis
Neurological syndromes
  Myelopathy from intrinsic or extrinsic processes
  Lumbosacral plexopathy, especially from diabetes
  Neuropathy, including inflammatory demyelinating type (i.e. Guillain–Barré)
  Mononeuropathy, including causalgia
  Myopathy, including myositis and metabolic causes

Referred pain
  Gastrointestinal disorders
  Genitourinary disorders, including nephrolithiasis, prostatitis and pyelonephritis
  Gynaecological disorders, including ectopic pregnancy and pelvic inflammatory disease
  Abdominal aortic aneurysm
  Hip pathology
Psychosocial causes
  Compensatable injury
  Somatoform pain disorder
  Psychiatric syndromes, including delusional pain
  Drug seeking
  Abusive relationships
  Seeking disability or out-of-work status

Unfortunately, some patients with sciatica secondary to nerve impingement syndromes at the nerve root level report muscle tenderness along with their radiculopathy. This can make diagnostic considerations particularly difficult. For a more in-depth review of these conditions the reader is referred to the textbook by Travell and Simons.[40]

Other muscle syndromes like fibromyalgia or chronic fatigue syndrome

Table 6.4 A simple classification for low back pain syndrome. (Adapted from Katz[36])

	Lifetime prevalence	Clinical features	Resolved at 3 months
Mechanical LBP	>80%	Non-specific ubiquitous Non-dermatomal radiation Worse with activity Neurological examination normal Often musculoskeletal in origin	90%
Herniated nucleus pulposus	40%	Peak incidence in forties Sciatic distribution Worse with Valsalva, flexion Monoradiculopathy on examination	60–80%
Spinal stenosis	NA	Peak incidence in elderly Broad distribution of symptoms Worse with extension Polyradiculopathy on examination	<10%
Chronic LBP	<1%	All ages Associated with psychological, social dysfunction Symptoms and disability dissociated from impairments	Variable course
Infection and tumours	NA	Pain constant No comfortable position Elevated sedimentation rate Systemic features	NA

LBP = low back pain; NA = not available.

Table 6.5 Quebec Task Force Classification on Spinal Disorders. (Reproduced from reference[37])

Pain without radiation
Pain plus radiation to proximal extemity
Pain plus radiation to distal extremity
Pain plus radiation to extremity plus neurological signs
Nerve root compression suggested by radiograph (e.g. listhesis)
Nerve root compression confirmed by imaging (CT, MRI, myelography)
Spinal stenosis
Postsurgical (1–6 months postoperatively)
Postsurgical (>6 months postoperatively)
Chronic pain syndrome
Other diagnoses

Duration characterised as <7 days, 7 days to 7 weeks, or >7 weeks.
Work status at evaluation noted as working or idle.

144

can produce low back pain symptoms.[41] However, these syndromes should produce diffuse symptoms in other regions of the body which separates them from other aetiologies of low back pain.

Degenerative disc disease

The role of the intervertebral disc in the production of low back pain continues in controversy. Certainly, degenerative disc disease produces many of the symptoms of mechanical low back pain.[42–45] The injection of saline or contrast material into a degenerative disc often produces radicular pain which is familiar to the patient.[46] Intervertebral discs begin to degenerate some time in the third decade of life, yet most do not produce painful symptoms. Why a minority of these discs produce debilitating back pain is not presently clear.

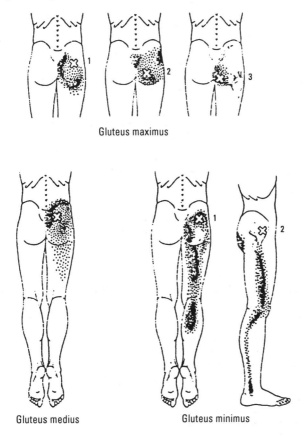

Fig 6.2 Trigger points (×) and referred pain patterns from the gluteus maximus, medius and minimus muscles. Note the radicular pattern of pain referral. (Adapted from Travell and Simons[40])

145

Facet arthropathy

Universal agreement does not exist on whether derangements of the facet joint produce complaints of low back pain. The inconsistency and non-specific signs and symptoms which have been reported in patients with facet pain have been used as evidence against a real facet syndrome.[47]

The facet joint is richly innervated with contributions coming from at least two nerves.[48-50] Many investigators believe that these joints do produce pain either with or without radicular symptomatology.[51 52] Unfortunately, there has not been any good method of confirming whether the joint is generating the pain complaint without performing an invasive diagnostic block. Conflicting evidence exists concerning the ability of a diagnostic block to predict the efficacy of a confirmatory block in relieving a patient's pain complaint.[53]

In summary, derangements of the facet joint most likely produce pain. Whether the symptoms and signs which result from facet disease are consistent enough to label this a syndrome is much less clear, and the efficacy of treatment options must be considered carefully in this group of patients.

Sacroiliac joint disease

The sacroiliac joint is classified as a true diarthroidal (synovial) joint which may possess multiple innervations.[54-58] The smallness of the joint relative to the forces across it makes it susceptible to stress and injury. Stability of the joint is maintained by a complex series of ligaments.

The varying innervation of this joint may account for the different pain presentations which can occur with joint pathology. Pain is most commonly located posteriorly over the joint although radiation into the buttocks is common. Further radiation into the posterior thigh also occurs while further radiation below the knee is extremely unlikely. The referred pain pattern does not follow a true radicular pattern which differentiates sacroiliac pain from sciatica. It has been reported that the pain can radiate into the groin.

The natural history of sacroiliac joint disease is unknown. Differences of opinion exist concerning the incidence of low back pain from disturbances within the sacroiliac joint. The joint is believed to undergo arthrofibrosis as a person ages. This limits active motion of the joint in the older patient and should make the joint less susceptible to producing low back pain symptoms.

Vertebral disc herniation

Lumbar vertebral disc herniation occurs most frequently (>95%) at the L4-5 and L5-S1 levels.[4 59] Herniation of the disc does not invariably cause pain as demonstrated by patients who have findings of herniation on MRI yet have no pain.[60][61] The pain which does result from a herniated disc is believed to come from either mechanical and/or chemical irritation of the respective nerve root. Depending on the size and location of the herniation either mechanical forces of the herniated segment onto the nerve root or chemical irritation from extravasated contents of the disc onto the nerve root produces irritation of the involved nerve.

Herniation of the L4–5 nerve root produces pain in the low back which radiates down the buttocks, posterior thigh, anterolateral leg, medial foot and great toe. Herniation of the L5–S1 nerve root produces similar pain except the distal referral pattern extends to the lateral leg, lateral foot and lateral toes. Pain complaints should always correlate with radiographic findings. If they do not correlate, one should be suspicious that a different pain generator is responsible for the patient's complaints.

Spinal stenosis

Spinal stenosis is classified as either congenital (rare) or acquired, and involves narrowing of either the spinal canal (central stenosis) or neural foramen (foraminal stenosis).[36] Acquired spinal stenosis is most commonly degenerative in nature and progressive. Degenerative spinal stenosis produces cauda equina impingement through osteophyte formation, hypertrophied ligamentum flavum, hypertrophied facets, protrusion of disc material and/or degenerative listhesis.[62][63]

The natural history of spinal stenosis normally follows a progressive course. Many patients eventually require surgical decompression although time from onset of first back pain symptoms to surgery is extremely variable and has been reported to vary from less than 1 month to 33+ years.[64][65] Hallmark symptoms include bilateral leg pain with walking which is relieved by rest and anteroflexion of the spine.

Numbness along with pain in the lower extremities during ambulation have caused this symptom to be termed pseudoclaudication since it resembles vascular claudication.[66][67] Arterial pulses are normal in spinal stenotic patients. A polyradicular pain pattern exists which is classically exacerbated with lumbar extension.

Spondylolisthesis

Spondylolisthesis is defined as displacement of one vertebral body on the next. This can occur in either a posterior or anterior direction. In the lumbar region displacement almost always occurs in the anterior direction. Minor slippage is rarely believed to cause pain and has been estimated to occur in 10–15% of elderly patients.[59] Acute pain can occur from stretch of the anterior and posterior longitudinal ligaments. Marked slippage of 75–100% of the vertebrae can produce radicular symptoms and occasionally bowel and bladder symptoms.[5][59]

The natural history of spondylolisthesis was originally believed to produce progressive symptoms and continued slippage.[68 69] Recent studies have suggested that the risk of progression is small (approximately 10%) even in young patients.[70–72] Mild malalignment does not necessarily infer spinal instability. If pain is exacerbated by movement, short term bracing has been recommended.[59]

Lumbar arachnoiditis

Lumbar arachnoiditis occurs most frequently in the patient who has had prior surgery or other invasive procedures to the spinal canal (e.g. myelography).[59 73] In the low back, scarring and thickening of the leptomeninges within the subarachnoid space produces inflammation of the nerve roots within the cauda equina.[74]

The pain of arachnoiditis is commonly experienced in either a non-dermatomal or multi-dermatomal pattern. Magnetic resonance imaging reveals either:

1 Peripheral matting of the nerve roots and the appearance of an empty dural sac
2 A central conglomeration of nerve roots
3 A soft tissue mass which replaces the subarachnoid space.[59 74]

The natural history does not usually produce resolution of the scarring. Inflammation of the nerves is not felt to be present in later stages which can produce a decrease in pain symptoms. Surgical lysis of adhesions has not often been successful in relieving symptoms as further adhesions replace those lysed.

Failed low back syndrome

This term is usually reserved for patients who have recalcitrant pain following one or more operations on the low back.[73 75 76] This syndrome is also termed post laminectomy syndrome, and the pain complaints are most likely multifactorial in origin. Arachnoiditis certainly produces the complaints of low back pain in some of these patients. Poor patient selection for surgery has been cited as possibly the major factor in producing this group of patients.[77 78] An analysis of 102 patients who underwent repeated surgical procedures demonstrated that poor patient selection was more common than technical surgical failure.[79] Other causes of failed back surgery include inadequate diagnosis, inadequate surgical decompression, recurrent disc herniation, secondary instability and direct surgical trauma.[75 76]

Pain can occur in this group of patients secondary to severe deconditioning of the lower back muscles. In patients whose pain complaints begin after a reasonable postsurgical pain-free interval, further diagnostic workup should be performed to try and isolate the cause of pain. If the pain generator can be isolated, specific treatment can be offered to help ameliorate symptoms.

Systemic and rheumatological aetiologies

Systemic causes of low back pain need to be considered in patients who present with low back symptoms. The most common causes of systemic disorders include malignancy and infection.[80][81] Primary bony tumours of the vertebral column are rare, but metastatic disease, particularly from breast, prostate and lung, occur frequently.

Infectious causes of low back pain include osteomyelitis and epidural abscess. The incidence of tuberculosis has rebounded in some populations and should be considered when other infectious aetiologies have been eliminated. Treatment for infectious causes of low back pain should begin as soon as confirmation is made. These systemic aetiologies provide further evidence that the astute clinician should never discount low back pain as mechanical, non-descript or unimportant for finding the diagnosis and pain generator.

Rheumatological disorders most likely to produce low back pain include ankylosing spondylitis, osteoporosis, degenerative osteoarthritis, myofascial pain syndrome and fibromyalgia.[59] Diagnosis is confirmed with the appropriate radiographic and laboratory testing. Medical management follows as indicated.

Diagnostic evaluation

History

Obtaining an accurate and thorough history from the patient is essential to making the correct diagnosis.[5][6][33] Associated signs and symptoms with aetiologies of low back pain are shown in Table 6.6.[73] The practitioner should determine early in the interview if the patient is experiencing an initial episode of low back pain or a recurrence of previous problems. A new onset of low back pain without an inciting incident in an older individual should raise a suspicion of metastatic disease.

A history of trauma is often encountered in the patient with mechanical low back pain. This can occur as a single event or a result of repetitive events. Occupational factors are important in patients who do prolonged or repetitive lifting. Since the epidemiology of most episodes of low back pain has found natural resolution of symptoms within 4 weeks, knowledge of the duration of symptoms aids greatly in understanding the likelihood of the episode progressing to a chronic state.

Factors which aggravate or relieve symptoms provide clues to the aetiology of the pain. Patients with mechanical low back pain, herniated

Table 6.6 Signs and symptoms: causes of low back pain. (Reproduced from Walker and Cousins[73])

	Facet joint	Instability	Myogenic	Hernia disc	Arachnoiditis	Spinal stenosis
Paravertebral pain	+ +	+	+ +	±	±	−
Paravertebral tenderness	+ +	+	+ +	±	±	−
Midspinal pain	−	+ +	+	−	±	−
Midspinal tenderness	−	+ +	+	−	±	−
Pain increased by motion	Hyperext/ rotation	Flex	+	Hyperext/ rotation	±	Hyperext/ walking
Pain relieved on flexion	−	−	−	−	−	+ +
Neurological deficit	−	−	−	+ +	±	Walking
Tension signs	−	−	(Spine)	+ +	+ +	−
Electrophysiology	−	−	−	+ +	+	+ +
Diagnostic imaging	−	CT	−	MRI/CT	MRI	MRI/CT

discs, spinal stenosis, facet arthropathy or spondylolisthesis can usually find a position which relieves their symptoms. However, patients with systemic causes of low back pain (e.g. tumour or infection) often are unable to achieve relief. Patients with herniated discs often find lumbar extension more comfortable, while patients with spinal stenosis can enlarge the cross-sectional area of the spinal canal and obtain relief of symptoms in a lumbar flexion position.

Patients with herniated discs often report numbness in addition to their pain, and aggravation of symptoms with sneezing, cough or other Valsalva manoeuvres. While it has been reported that radicular symptoms in the L5–S1 distribution have a sensitivity of 85% and a specificity of 88% for herniated discs, this is probably related to the population of patients examined.[33 62] Most chronic pain clinics see patients with radiculopathies who do not have disc herniations as a cause of their low back pain symptoms.

Patients with spinal stenosis and spondylolisthesis often report aggravation of their symptoms with ambulation. The general pain reported with spinal stenosis is not usually dermatomal, as seen with disc protrusion. Facet arthropathy symptoms are often improved with lumbar flexion, a manoeuvre which offloads the facet joint. Classically, patients who have mechanical low back pain notice a worsening of symptoms with exercise while patients with inflammatory aetiologies will note an improvement.

The history of patients with low back pain should include questions concerning the psychosocial impact of the pain episode. Many studies have demonstrated the association of the low back pain with psychosocial disturbances.[16 18 19] This is particularly true in patients with chronic symptoms (>6 months) and those who have litigation or disability issues ongoing. Most patients who have symptoms which are not easily explained by organic pathology and/or have had symptoms beyond an expected duration should be strongly considered for psychological screening and therapy when indicated.

Physical examination

The physical examination of the patient with low back pain should be thorough, systematic, and include inspection, palpation and movements of the patient which reproduce the pain and help confirm an aetiology to the symptoms. With inspection of the back the examiner often sees pelvic asymmetry, poor vertebral alignment, poor posture and/or loss of lumbar lordosis. These conditions are common in patients with mechanical low back pain.

Palpation of the patient should include all muscles of the low back and buttocks. Palpation of trigger points commonly reproduce radicular symptoms in patients with myofascial pain syndromes. Some patients with disc protrusions will experience muscle spasms in the low back, which, on examination, may appear as trigger points. Further testing is indicated in these patients.

Lumbar flexion is diminished in many patients with low back pain and does not exclude many diagnoses. Patients presenting with reproduction of radicular symptoms during reduced flexion alert the examiner to disc protrusion. In contrast, facet arthropathy produces increased pain for many patients during lumbar extension. This is presumed to occur secondary to loading of the facet during extension. Pain with rotation of the spine and lateral bending is also considered a non-specific sign of facet disease.

When nerve root pathology exists the physical examination should provide evidence of which root(s) are involved. Sensory abnormalities of the lower extremity should be carefully mapped for dermatomal accuracy (Fig. 6.3). While dermatomes of the lower extremity exhibit more interpatient variability than the upper extremity, the lack of dermatomal specificity should alert the examiner to other possible causes of sensory hyperaesthesia. Motor weakness, when present should correlate with sensory findings.

The specificity of motor findings has greatly outweighed those seen with sensory abnormalities.[33] Reflexes are equally important, with the ankle reflex confirmatory evidence of pathology to the S1 root and the patellar reflex used to test the L4 root. No reflex pathway tests for L5 disease.

The straight leg examination tests the effect of stretch on an inflamed nerve root. Thus, patients who have an injured nerve root in the L4, L5 or S1 distribution would be expected to show reproduction of symptoms with stretch of the root. The patient should be positioned supine and the lower extremity raised with the knee fully extended. The test is considered positive only if radicular pain is reproduced in the appropriate distribution with elevation of the extremity at 60 degrees or less. Further pain is elucidated if the foot is dorsiflexed. Pain in the back or back of the thigh is recorded as a negative result. Further confirmatory evidence for nerve root involvement is found if elevation of the contralateral lower extremity reproduces the patient's pain.

The physical examination also helps to differentiate organic from non-organic pathology. Few patients are sophisticated enough to fool an experienced examiner. Inconsistencies in the physical examination should be explored fully to try and explain their appearance. Those patients whose

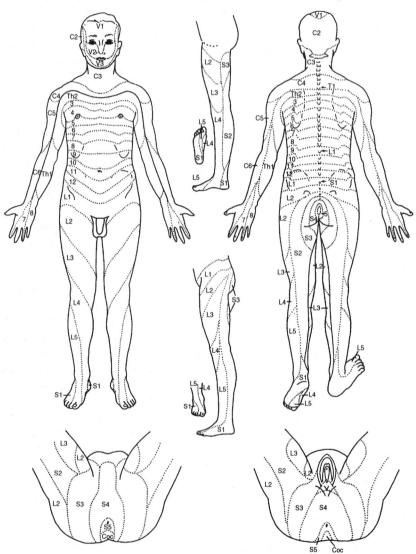

Fig 6.3

152

physical examination points to non-organic aetiologies should be referred to a multidisciplinary pain centre for psychological evaluation and pain management.

Laboratory evaluation

Laboratory evaluation is not routinely indicated for patients who present with low back pain. If a patient is suspected of having a rheumatological disorder an erythrocyte sedimentation rate should be done as a screening test. HLA-B27 antigen testing is not routinely indicated, since the antigen is found in around 6% of the population, while less than 1% of the population has ankylosing spondylitis.[82] A complete white blood cell count with differential is indicated if infection is suspected.

Radiography

The use of radiography is considered controversial in the evaluation of the patient with low back pain. Despite its continued use, several studies have not demonstrated any advantage of routine lumbar spine films in the average patient with low back pain.[34 83] There has been a poor correlation between the abnormalities seen on plain films and patient symptoms.[34 84–86]

In a large retrospective analysis 75% of patients had radiographs which were either normal or had no clinical significance.[87] Oblique views added useful information in only 2·7% of patients examined.[4 88] Selection criteria have been proposed for when to order plain lumbar X-rays.[34] Using these criteria in 621 patients, all patients with malignant disease were found by X-ray examination, as were 13 of 14 patients with fractures.[34]

Magnetic resonance imaging, CT, and myelography are frequently utilised in the evaluation of patients with suspected herniated discs. Unfortunately, they are expensive tests and should be ordered judiciously for cases where therapy can be directed by the findings. It must also be remembered that approximately 20% of asymptomatic patients have herniated discs or spinal stenosis on MRI or CT[89–91] (Table 6.7).

Disagreement exists over which test best evaluates the patient with low back pain. MRI allows for better visualisation of more structures in the low back, including morphological and biochemical sequelae of intervertebral disc degeneration, facet disease, malignant involvement, nerve root impingement, spinal stenosis and spondylolisthesis. In a recent review of the benefits of MRI it was cautioned that "substantial percentages of asymptomatic people have abnormal lumbosacral MRI studies". This demands accurate correlation of MRI to the clinical situation.

Myelography and myelography-enhanced CT are believed by some to provide better images of nerve roots and pathology surrounding the nerve root. While the morbidity of myelography (arachnoiditis) has greatly

Table 6.7 Prevalence of bulges, protrusions and extrusions on MRI scans in 98 asymptomatic subjects and 27 symptomatic subjects. (Adapted from Wipf and Deyo[5] and Jensen, et al[91])

	Subjects					
	Bulge		Protrusion		Extrusion	
	No	%	No	%	No	%
Evaluator 1						
Asymptomatic subjects	52	53	30	31	2	2
Symptomatic subjects	23	85	14	52	8	30
Evaluator 2						
Asymptomatic subjects	50	51	23	23	0	
Symptomatic subjects	18	67	15	56	6	22
Average of the two evaluators						
Asymptomatic subjects	51	52	26·5	27	1	1
Symptomatic subjects	20·5	76	14·5	54	7	26

diminished with the development of water-soluble, non-ionic contrast, these invasive tests should be performed only when specific indications exist.

Discography

MRI, CT and myelography provide static images of potential pathology in the low back. They do not provide direct information which could be used to correlate the radiographic finding and the patient's pain. These procedures are also limited in their ability to visualise a disc which has not protruded or herniated.

Discography has been advocated as a method to evaluate discs in a dynamic fashion.[92-94] It is believed that discs can possess internal derangements such as annular fissures or radial tears which are commonly not visualised by MRI. The invasiveness of discography makes it inappropriate for visualisation of routine disc herniation.

Injection of saline or contrast into a damaged and painful disc must reproduce the patient's pain for the diagnostic discogram to be considered positive. If injection causes no pain or does not replicate the patient's familiar pain, then the discogram should be considered negative regardless of the morphological appearance of the disc. This is validated by the presence of many degenerated discs which do not produce pain. Following injection of contrast, CT imaging is performed within 4 hours to best visualise the discs in question.

Several studies have examined the usefulness of discography.[95-97] Opponents of discography claim that abnormal discograms result only in unnecessary surgery. The only surgical option for patients with intrinsically abnormal, painful discs is surgical stabilisation.[98] Whether this procedure in this population of patients produces relief of symptoms is debated.[99]

If discography is used as a diagnostic test it is probably only indicated in very select cases where other diagnostic tests have been inconclusive. Determining a disc as the pain generator may be useful information for the patient, even if surgical correction is not an option. Repeat testing and examinations may be avoided once the disc is implicated as the cause of pain.

Diagnostic selective nerve block procedures

Following the complete history, physical examination and radiographic testing, a clear diagnosis will still be lacking in some patients. If the need to locate the patient's pain generator is still desired, selective nerve blocks can be performed to help confirm a diagnosis. The most commonly performed diagnostic nerve blocks include the facet block, differential spinal or epidural and a selective nerve root block.

The facet block has been advocated as a diagnostic block because of the difficulty in performing direct examination of the facet joint.[100 101] The history and physical examination often provide non-specific positive findings for facet disease. Radiogaphic examination often finds facet pathology, but studies have demonstrated that patients with degenerative facets by X-ray can be asymptomatic.[47] A very active debate continues as to the diagnostic validity of facet syndrome and/or the ability to alter the course of facet disease with nerve block techniques.[47 102] It does seem probable that the facet joint can play a significant role as a pain generator in the low back, and patients could benefit diagnostically from this information.[103-105]

Selective nerve root blocks have been employed when other tests have failed to conclusively identify a particular nerve root as the aetiology for a patient's pain. This occurs in patients whose pain may not fit a traditional dermatomal pattern or when the intraspinal pathology is sufficiently complex to hinder knowledge of what is producing the pain. Isolating a nerve root and anaesthetising it with a small amount of concentrated local anaesthetic provides confirmatory evidence of its role as the patient's pain generator. It should be cautioned that temporary relief of pain by a selective nerve root does not ensure that surgical decompression or other treatment modality (e.g. selective steroid nerve root injection) can effectively resolve the pain.

Differential spinal and epidural blocks have often been advocated in patients with sympathetic pain syndromes, even though their ability to selectively block the sympathetic nerves has not been well established. These blocks can provide selected information for some patients who have radicular low back pain.

Patients who have neuropathic conditions and pain which has centralised will not derive pain relief during a differential block, despite a complete local anaesthetic block at the spinal cord level. This can be extremely useful information as these patients would not be expected to derive pain relief from surgical decompression or other therapy at the spinal cord level. A differential central neuraxial block can also be used to determine placebo responders. In addition, this information can be used to help guide therapeutic choices. The reader is referred to other texts for more complete information on techniques of the differential block.[106]

Therapeutic interventions

Management options for patients with low back pain include medical regimens, exercise programmes, medical psychology, surgery, and multidisciplinary pain programmes. As stated at the beginning of this chapter, most patients who experience low back pain do not require specific intervention as symptoms spontaneously resolve within 2–4 weeks. The challenge is identifying those patients whose symptoms do not resolve and administer therapy in a timely and cost-efficient fashion. Delays in therapy, particularly in the worker who is on disability, may predispose to a prolongation of time spent on disability.

Outcome studies

Many treatment regimens for low back pain patients have not been subjected to good, prospective outcome studies. Management is too often empirical and based on anecdotal experience. Chronic low back pain is often multifactorial in nature, and the management is complex. Well-designed, prospective, randomised, blinded multicentre trials need undertaking to help delineate which therapies are helpful for what subsets of patients.

Outcome studies have examined the 'natural' history of certain populations of low back pain patients. Particular attention has been directed to the patient who has had recurrent back episodes and lost work secondary to low back pain.[107–110] A direct negative correlation exists between length of time out of work and the likelihood of returning to work. Identifying those patients at risk of staying out of work on disability represents the initial step at prevention of disability. The most effective early treatment for these "at risk" patients has yet to be defined based on outcome criteria.

Outcomes for surgical procedures for different low back pain populations have been conflicting.[107 111 112] Intense rehabilitation programmes have shown benefit in some populations of patients (Gross, personal communication).[113] At the University of Miami Comprehensive Pain and Rehabilitation Center (UMCPRC), patients who underwent a 4-week intensive inpatient treatment programme had greater return to work rates and used less healthcare services (e.g. physician services, hospitalisations, and surgeries) than their counterparts. Intense outpatient multidisciplinary programmes have also been popular with chronic low back pain patients.

Medical management

Whether medications can alter the outcome of low back pain is unknown. They certainly provide relief of symptoms in some patients and may allow other patients to engage in physical therapy activities and other programmes which may alter outcome. Medications have also been argued to hinder patients' recovery via side-effects, problems with addiction, and the promotion of a disability lifestyle. When used, medications should be administered judiciously with appropriate follow-up and a clear understanding by the practitioner and patient of the benefits/risks of any drug prescribed.

Non-steroidal anti-inflammatory drugs (NSAIDs)

Table 6.8 shows many of the more commonly used NSAIDs for low back pain. Anti-inflammation has been the physiological basis for their use, although inflammation may not be present in many conditions of chronic low back pain. NSAIDs have also enjoyed popularity among practitioners because of their low addiction potential.

Efficacy should be monitored closely when NSAIDs are used. They can be given daily or as "prn" (as needed) drugs. These drugs can be particularly effective following physical therapy or other activities which might induce inflammation. If one is not effective a second drug in a different class should be trialled. If several trials have been unsuccessful NSAIDs should be discontinued.

Risks of NSAIDs have been underappreciated by many practitioners. Gastrointestinal bleeding produces the greatest morbidity from NSAIDs. Patients on chronic NSAIDs, some of whom derive only marginal benefits from their use, can develop significant gastrointestinal bleeds resulting in hospitalisations and subsequent invasive procedures. Renal toxicity can lead to renal insufficiency and rarely to renal failure. Renal failure occurs most commonly in the NSAID misuser.

Table 6.8   Representative list of NSAIDs useful for low back pain

Propionic acids	Carboxylic acid
Ibuprofen (Motrin)	Etodolac (Lodine)
Flurbiprofen (Ansaid)	Ketorolac (Toradol)
Keptoprofen (Orudis)	Salicylates
Naproxen (Naprosyn)	Diflunisal (Dolobid)
Naproxen sodium (Aleve)	Salsalate (Disalcid)
Oxaprozin (DayPro)	Choline magnesium trisalicylate (Trilisate)
Fenoprofen (Nalfon)	Oxicams
Anthranilic acids	Piroxicams (Feldene)
Sulindac (Clinoril)	Naphthylalkalone
Indomethacin (Indocin)	Nabumtone (Relafen)
Tolmetin (Tolectin)	
Phenylacetic acid	
Diclofenac sodium (Voltaren)	
Diclofenac potassium (Cataflam)	

Antidepressants

The association of chronic low back pain and depression is well chronicled.[114-116] It is less clear whether depression precedes the progression of intermittent back pain episodes to a chronic pain state, or follows. One can certainly understand how disabled patients living with chronic pain would experience a reactive depression.

Because the association between chronic low back pain and depression is closely linked it becomes equally difficult to understand if the benefits realised from antidepressant medication result from treatment of the pain or depression. While the literature has been somewhat contradictory, many articles have found the antidepressant medications do provide analgesia for a variety of chronic pain syndromes.[117-120]

A review of six placebo-controlled studies have examined the benefit of antidepressant medications on chronic low back.[121] Only one of three articles found antidepressants (imipramine) superior in the relief of pain. One of three studies found an antidepressant superior to placebo on affecting functional disability, and no study showed an antidepressant superior to placebo in the management of depression. The authors of the review concluded that all of the studies suffered from serious methodological flaws which precluded a meta-analysis and mandated a need for further, better designed studies.

Muscle relaxants

Muscle spasm produces much of the pain seen in chronic low back pain. The erector spinalis, multifidus, psoas, quadratus lumborum, gluteals, and piriformis muscles are all large muscles which have a significant role in movements of the back and hip. The stresses and strains placed on these muscles with bending, lifting, etc. make them susceptible to injury. Abnormalities of the spine such as scoliosis place particular strain on these muscles to compensate for this asymmetry.

An overused or traumatically injured muscle is susceptible to spasm and becoming chronically contracted. A muscle relaxant which could allow the muscle to relax and stretch to a normal resting length would be very beneficial. Unfortunately, muscle relaxants in current practice do not have a direct effect on voluntary muscles of the body. Their action is through the CNS and may not produce true relaxation of the muscle itself. The efficacy of this class of medication has been lacking in scientific studies. However, clinical experience may support their use in select patients. One should watch for sedative side-effects and attempt to document that patients are receiving relief of symptoms that allow improved function.

Nerve membrane stabilisers

Antiepileptic medications have been frequently employed in patients with nerve injury. This class of agents has the ability to raise the membrane depolarisation threshold through their effect on the sodium conduction channel. Their use in low back pain should be reserved for patients who have documented evidence of nerve injury. This predominantly occurs from injury to a nerve root within the spinal canal, such as from a herniated nucleus pulposus.

The correct dose of medication in this class may differ from the antiseizure dose. It is best to titrate the dose of medicine to the desired effect. Escalation of dose is considered appropriate as long as side-effects can be avoided. Maximal analgesic benefit can be expected within 2–4 weeks from when the patient reaches a therapeutic level.

Opiates

The use of opiates in the management of low back pain continues to provoke an emotional debate which is often not founded on good scientific evidence. The main argument for opiate use is the fact that this class of analgesics can provide significant pain relief in a large percentage of low back pain patients. This may allow patients to engage in important rehabilitative programmes and return to a functional lifestyle. Those against opiate use appropriately look at the highly addictive nature of opiates, the tolerance they can produce in many patients with subsequent need for dose escalation, and the lack of studies to support any benefit beyond short term pain relief.

This author's clinical experience with chronic low back pain patients has been positive, although many caveats exist. Patients such as those with failed back surgery and arachnoiditis for whom few other options exist can benefit from opiates. Some of these patients do not show dose escalation, maintain analgesic benefit, and return to productive lifestyles.

Many patients cannot manage opiate medication appropriately. Either dose escalation becomes a significant problem or an addictive personality precludes effective use of these medications. If a pain clinic decides to use opiates in chronic non-malignant pain, they can assure themselves of attracting a disproportionate number of opiate-seeking patients. Formal, written opiate contracts and a firm understanding of the patient's responsibility in managing these medications helps circumvent some problems.

Which opiate should be used in chronic pain is also frequently debated. Potency differs between opiates and some patients do not require strong opiates in the management of their pain. For most patients use of an opiate which allows a long dosing interval is preferable to frequent repeat administrations. Some patients have episodic or intermittent pain patterns whereby a short-acting opiate may be appropriate. If dose escalation does not occur and total daily dose remains acceptable, then change to a long-acting opiate can be avoided.

The author's experience has found that the patients who respond best to

Table 6.9   Ideal non-cancer pain patient for opiate management

Pathophysiological processes clear and definitive e.g. arachnoiditis versus fibromyalgia
Psychological issues minimal e.g. reactive depression versus symptom exaggeration
Patient is working or functional or desire to achieve these goals is evaluated and believed
sincere opinion: pain relief, as a goal, is secondary
Motivated, responsible patient will adhere to contract

opiates have characteristics listed in Table 6.9. Treatment issues are shown in Table 6.10. If breakthrough medications are required, non-narcotic adjuvants should be stressed. Written contracts are essential and the pain practitioner should keep good documentation of prescriptions written and any patient discrepancies.

Methadone has proved an excellent agent for many patients with low back pain who require an opiate. Patients who respond to low dose (20–30 mg/day) seem to maintain analgesic effect without subsequent dose escalation better than those who require larger doses. Opiates which have been manufactured in controlled-release preparations such as morphine and oxycodone have also been used. Clinical practice states that controlled-release preparations produce less problems with dose escalation, euphoria, and addiction.

Physical therapy

Physical therapy has been considered by most multidisciplinary pain centres as a cornerstone therapy for patients with chronic low back pain. Classic teaching to bed rest a back injury for 6 weeks produced many deconditioned patients who subsequently required weeks to restrengthen to their prior state.[122] While it remains unclear when a patient should begin aggressive exercises and activities following an injury, bed rest is rarely indicated.

It is beyond the scope of this chapter to provide detailed information on different aspects of physical therapy activities, and the reader is referred to an excellent review of Koes concerning the benefits and pitfalls of physiotherapy.[123] It has become less fashionable to use time-honoured modalities such as massage, hot/cold packs or electrical stimulation. Outcome data have not demonstrated benefit from these techniques

Table 6.10   Treatment issues in non-cancer opiate management

Written contract essential to success
Careful documentation in the chart
Use long-lasting agents which employ infrequent dosing intervals
Use single drug regimens in majority of patients—utilise non-narcotic adjuvants for
   breakthrough pain
Short-acting agents appropriate for patient with infrequent analgesic needs and when dose
   escalation has not been a problem
Avoid agents with significant euphoria

although in select patients these modalities, when used in short courses, allow for earlier involvement in exercise programmes and other restorative programmes.

Exercise and reconditioning programmes which stress functional restoration may provide the best therapy for a majority of low back patients.[113 124] These should be individualised to meet the patient's specific needs. Progression to home programmes is always the goal, with the understanding that these exercises should become a daily routine, often for the rest of the patient's life.

Medical psychology

Acute and chronic low back pain differ immensely in the likelihood of concurrent psychological issues which affect recovery. Most sufferers of chronic low back pain experience some reactive depression as they struggle to accept living with a chronic condition. For others depression becomes a severe problem which impacts the patient's pain in a major way.

While no specific psychological profile has been assigned to the patient with chronic low back pain, the identification and diagnosis of mental pathology should be a major effort of any comprehensive low back pain programme. There may not be economic justification to have all patients evaluated by a licensed psychologist in the present medical environment. However, present screening tests can be administered in a cost-efficient manner which helps the psychologically untrained physician to know which patients might benefit from psychological intervention.

A screening test which is both easy to administer and straightforward in its interpetation is the Symptom Checklist-90 (SCL-90). The Beck Depression Inventory (BVI) has also been utilised by centres in the screening of patients with low back pain. More extensive tests such as the Minnesota Multiphasic Personality Inventory are not indicated as screening devices for several reasons. They are costly, require significant time to administer and score, and provide substantial information which is unnecessary or unwarranted for many patients. Certainly, these tests have a place in the diagnostic workup and management of some patients.

Nerve blocks

The role of nerve blocks in the management of low back pain has several facets. The majority of blocks are designed to be therapeutic. Equally beneficial are some blocks which provide diagnostic information. Nerve blocks can be used effectively to provide valuable information about where the specific pain generator is located. Since presenting signs and symptoms of low back pain can be non-specific, this information proves essential and often unobtainable by any other test.

The efficacy of nerve blocks for chronic low back pain, as measured by outome studies, has been slow to evolve. While many practitioners discuss

161

the benefits of these procedures the scientific evidence is lacking. Negative studies have also been infrequent. This lack of well-controlled, randomised studies makes specific treatment recommendations difficult in some cases. Also, in today's medico-economic environment the pain community needs to demonstrate the benefit of the treatments and services they provide. Hopefully, these studies are forthcoming.

Myoneural nerve blocks

Some of the largest muscles of the body are found in the low back region. These muscles help to keep us erect and allow us to move in a variety of ways. Injury to these muscles is undisputed; how they respond to trauma and why some patients develop chronic low back symptoms after injury is less clear. One treatment modality for low back pain of musculoskeletal origin is the injection of painful trigger points.

Different studies have examined the benefit of myoneural nerve blocks in chronic low back.[125–127] Some studies have demonstrated no difference between dry needling of trigger points and the injection of analgesic substances.[127] Other studies have reported marked improvement after the injection of local anaesthetics and/or corticosteroids.[126]

Common musculoskeletal sites for trigger points in the low back include the gluteal, erector spinae, quadratus lumborum and piriformis muscles. A knowledge of the referral patterns for these muscles and how to examine for their presence is essential prior to appropriate injection. The injection of trigger points should be performed based on the pain referral pattern and physical examination. Using small gauge needles (e.g. 25 gauge) is advised, and length is determined by the size of the patient and the muscles injected. A combination of bupivacaine 0·75% (for sensory analgesia), etidocaine 1% (for prolonged motor block) and dexamethasone (4 mg/10 ml, for anti-inflammation) is used in the author's institution. An upper limit of 0·3 ml/kg is advised.

Facet nerve block

The extensive innervation of the facet joint makes denervation an attractive option for the relief of low back pain. Different options exist for facet denervation. One can inject directly into the joint with either local anaesthetic, corticosteroid, or a neurolytic agent. Denervation can also be performed with either cryotherapy or radiofrequency techniques. Entering the joint with a needle can be difficult or impossible when significant hypertrophy is present. Furthermore, it is unclear whether it is preferable to inject the joint or block the sinuvertebral nerves to the joint. If the joint is injected small volumes are indicated (0·5–1·5 ml), since larger volumes can rupture the joint.

The most common nerve blocked to the facet joint is the median branch of the sinuvertebral or posterior rami nerve. As demonstrated in Fig. 6.4 this nerve is blocked by placing a needle into the "eye of the Scottie dog".[128]

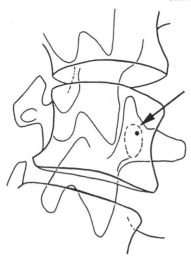

Fig 6.4 Cartoon description of the relationship of the lumbar facet joint and the "Scottie dog". Needle location (arrow) for block of the median branch nerve to the facet. The needle is positioned in the eye of the "Scottie dog". (Reproduced from Kline[128])

Following confirmation with X-ray, local anaesthetic with corticosteroid (2–3 ml with 20 mg depomedrol) is injected. If the patient derives benefit but has recurrence of symptoms, more permanent denervation may be indicated. This can be performed with either radiofrequency or cryo-analgesia. Radiofrequency tends to produce a more permanent lesion and utilises a probe which is easier to place into deep structures of the low back. Cryoanalgesia produces a block of intermediate duration.

Sacroiliac joint injection

The likelihood of the sacroiliac joint to produce pain has been debated. If physical examination and X-ray documentation suggest sacroiliac disease, the joint can be injected with a combination of local anaesthetic and corticosteroid. A more permanent block has been advocated with either phenol or radiofrequency.

Epidural steroid injection

The use of epidural steroid injections for low back pain should only follow careful history and physical examination. In equivocal cases radiological examination can help decide the likelihood of the patient deriving benefit from injection. Only patients who have inflammation of a nerve root(s) can expect to derive benefit from these injections.

No comparative studies have been performed with respect to corticosteroid preparations. Clearly agents such as Solu-Medrone, which contain high concentrations of benzyl alcohol, should be avoided. The two agents

163

which have been demonstrated safe when injected epidurally are triamcinolone and methylprednisolone in doses of 50–75 mg and 80–120 mg, respectively.[129] [130]

Both agents are commonly diluted in local anaesthetics before injection. While no studies have compared the efficacy of different volumes, 2–6 ml of bupivacaine 0·0625–0·25% are commonly used. If higher concentrations or volumes of bupivacaine are used patients must be checked closely for signs of motor block.

In patients who have had previous back surgery the best approach to the epidural space can be a difficult decision. Posterior fusions usually preclude entrance to the epidural space at the site of the fusion. While the epidural space can be found in patients who have undergone laminectomies, a higher incidence of inadvertent dural puncture must be accepted. This results primarily because the dura becomes adhered to the ligamentum flavum, completely obliterating the epidural space in some cases.

One should always try to place the epidural close to the intended site of action, therefore it is advantageous to place the epidural through the scar in some patients. This must be weighed against the obvious increased risk of dural puncture. If it is decided to avoid the scar the epidural can be placed either above the scar or via a caudal approach. If the caudal approach is performed a larger volume of local anaesthetic or saline (10–20 ml) is required to allow the corticosteroid to reach the site of action.

Patients with foraminal stenosis or isolated radiculopathy may benefit from selective nerve root injections of corticosteroids. This is best performed under fluoroscopic guidance. Inflamed, irritated nerve roots can be expected to derive the most benefit.

It is felt that some patients have significant nerve root irritation secondary to scar tissue in the epidural space. These patients may be candidates for epidural lysis of adhesions. It is recommended that the practitioner becomes thoroughly familiar with this technique and the possible complications before attempting it on patients. Hypertonic saline, when inadvertently injected intrathecally, can have catastrophic effects. Some patients after laminectomy may have scar tissue which obscures the free flow of CSF yet allows medication under positive pressure to theoretically enter the subarachnoid space. Strict adherence to the protocol should be routine and specific informed consent should be obtained. The reader is referred to other material for further information.[131]

Myeloscopy

Myeloscopy employs a fibreoptic scope which allows the operator the opportunity to look into the epidural space. The role of myeloscopy in the management of patients with low back pain is presently unclear. In theory the ability to direct corticosteroids directly to the involved nerve root(s) should produce more effective results.

164

Diagnostically, this modality should help define intraspinal pathology. Characteristics of the epidural space limit the size of the scope and may limit some of the therapeutic considerations such as direct visual lysis of adhesions. Anecdotal reports have been encouraging, although no controlled, randomised studies have been reported to date. Prospective studies are needed to help guide clinicians in the utility of this technique.

Spinal cord stimulation

The use of electrodes for stimulation of the posterior columns was reported many years ago.[132] Widespread clinical use of this concept waited for better technology which has been evolving over the past 10 years.[133–136] The present technology allows for a wide variety of options with posterior column stimulation. Specifically, 4–16 electrodes are presently advocated for patients with refractory axial low back pain and/or radiculopathy. These pain patterns can be stimulated in a vast number of permutations. The cost of complex systems is significant and merits careful screening prior to stimulation consideration.

Patients should be selected carefully for implantation. Highly motivated patients achieve the best results. All patients should be evaluated by a trained psychologist prior to an implantation trial. An excellent review of psychological considerations has been recently published.

The pain must be amenable to spinal cord stimulation. Patients who have significant radiculopathy in one lower extremity tend to respond better than patients whose pain is diffuse, with a significant low back component in the axial skeleton. All patients should receive a trial prior to permanent implantation. How long this trial should extend is currently debated. Two-week trials are not excessive, especially if results are equivocal. Trials up to 4 weeks are advocated by some practitioners (Krames, personal communication).

Provocative discography

It is beyond the scope of this chapter to review the controversy surrounding discography. This procedure is advocated as a dynamic test for investigating intrinsic disc pathology. It is not intended to replace CT or MRI scans which are superior in examining the presence of herniated discs. Intrinsically degenerative discs appear capable of producing pain and usually may not be discoverable by static tests such as MRI.

Provocative discography is considered a diagnostic test and not therapeutic. Opponents to discography argue accurately that there may not be specific treatment for intrinsically deranged discs, therefore discography has no utility. Certainly, fusions for positive discograms may not alter outcome. While some practitioners advocate radiofrequency lesioning in patients with painful, degenerative discs, the efficacy of this treatment is being evaluated. This should not limit provocative discography in select cases where an accurate diagnosis of the pain generator can save significant money in further diagnostic tests and prevent treatment that is not indicated.

The performance of discography must be done under strict protocol or the information obtained becomes useless. The risk of discography, predominantly discitis, is real, approaches 1%, and must be explained to the patient prior to the procedure. The reader is referred elsewhere for a specific outline of the protocol.[135]

Summary

The vast majority of people in all countries will experience an episode of low back pain. Fortunately, most recover with non-specific treatment, although recurrence may be high. Identifying risk factors and altering them wherever possible hopefully can decrease both the incidence and recurrence rates.

An extremely disproportionate amount of money is spent on the small percentage of patients who progress to chronic low back pain. Identifying the prognostic factors which affect the progression of acute low back pain to chronic low back pain hopefully can help decrease the likelihood of progression. Early intervention for those patients known to be at risk hopefully could alter the natural history of progression and save significant money in future care.

Treatment should be directed early to patients who do not respond to non-specific care. The use of directed, individualised treatment plans should help keep care affordable. Research, particularly outcome studies, needs to be performed to test different therapeutic strategies in an effort to change the present natural history of this very costly and debilitating problem.

References

1 Waddell G. A new clinical model for the treatment of low back pain. *Spine* 1987;**12**:632–44.
2 Frymoyer JW. Back pain and sciatica. *N Engl J Med* 1988;**318**:291–300.
3 Heliovarra M, Sievers K, Impivaaro O, *et al.* Descriptive epidemiology and public health aspects of low back pain. *Ann Med* 1989;**21**:327–33.
4 Mazanec DJ. Back pain: medical evaluation and therapy. *Cleve Clin J Med* 1995;**62**:163–8.
5 Wipf JE, Deyo RA. Low back pain. *Med Clin North Am* 1995;**79**:231–46.
6 Frymoyer JW. Predicting disability from low back pain. *Clin Orthop Rel Res* 1992;**279**:101.
7 Wheeler AH. Diagnosis and management of low back pain and sciatica. *Am Fam Physician* 1995;**52**:1333–41.
8 Frymoyer JW. Quality. An international challenge to the diagnosis and treatment of disorders of the lumbar spine. *Spine* 1993;**18**:2147–52.
9 Nachemson AL. *Low back pain. Causes, diagnosis and treatment.* Stockholm: The Swedish

Council of Technology Assessment in Health Care, 1991 (in Swedish).

10 Allan DB, Waddell G. A historical perspective on low back pain and disability. *Acta Orthop Scand* 1989;**234** (Suppl):1.

11 Bombardier C, Kerr MS, Shannon HS, *et al.* A guide to interpreting epidemiologic studies on the etiology of back pain. *Spine* 1994;**19**(18S):2047S–56S.

12 Nachemson AL. Newest knowledge of low back pain: a critical look. *Clin Orthop Rel Res* 1992;**279**:8–20.

13 Bergenudd H, Nilsson B. Back pain in middle age: occupational workload and psychologic factors. An epidemiologic study. *Spine* 1988;**13**:58.

14 Bigos SJ, Battie MC, Spengler DM, *et al.* A longitudinal, prospective study of industrial back injury reporting. *Clin Orthop* 1992;**279**:21.

15 Deyo RA, Diehl AK. Psychosocial predictors of disability in patients with low back pain. *J Rheumatol* 1988;**15**:1557.

16 Magora A. Investigation of the relation between low back pain and occupation. V Psychological aspects. *Scand J Rehabil Med* 1973;**5**:191.

17 Svensson HO, Andersson G. The relationship of low back pain, work history, work environment, and stress: a retrospective cross-sectional study of 38- to 64-year old women. *Spine* 1989;**14**:517.

18 Troup JDG, Foreman TK, Baxter CE, *et al.* The perception of back pain and the role of psychophysical tests of lifting capacity. *Spine* 1987;**12**:645.

19 Waddell G, Main CJ, Morris EW, *et al.* Chronic low back pain, psychologic distress, and illness behavior. *Spine* 1984;**9**:209.

20 Wolf HJ, Greenwood L, Pearson RJC. *Job satisfaction: a predictor of injury.* NIOSH, USA, 1989.

21 Deyo RA, Tsui-Wu YJ. Descriptive epidemiology of low back pain and its related medical care in the United States. *Spine* 1987;**12**:264.

22 Abenhaim L, Suissa S. Importance and economic burden of occupational back pain: a study of 2500 cases representative of Quebec. *J Occup Med* 1987;**29**:670.

23 Wood PHN, Bradley EM. Epidemiology of back pain. In: Jayson, MIV, III, ed, *The lumbar spine and back pain.* London: Churchill Livingstone, 1987:1–15.

24 Zuidema H. National statistics in the Netherlands. *Ergonomics* 1985;**28**:3.

25 Biering-Sorenson F, Thomsen C, Hilden J. Risk indicators for low back trouble. *Scand J Rehab Med* 1986;**21**:151–7.

26 Deyo RA, Bass JE. Lifestyle and low back pain. The influence of smoking and obesity. *Spine* 1989;**14**:501–6.

27 Kelsey JL, Githens PB, O'Connor T, *et al.* Acute prolapsed lumbar intervertebral disc. An epidemiologic study with special reference to driving automobiles and cigarette smoking. *Spine* 1984;**9**:608–13.

28 Bigos SJ, Battie MC, Spangler SM, *et al.* A prospective study of work perceptions and psychosocial factors affecting the report of back injury. *Spine* 1991;**16**:1–6.

29 Deyo RA, Tsui-Wui YJ. Functional disability due to back pain. A population-based study indicating the importance of socioeconomic factors. *Arthritis Rheum* 1987;**20**:1247–53.

30 Herzog RJ. CT. Clinical efficacy and outcome in the diagnosis and treatment of low back pain. In: Weinstein JN, ed, New York: Raven, 1992:67–89.

31 Svensson HO. Low back pain in forty to forty-seven year old men. II Socioeconomic factors and previous sickness absence. *Scand J Rehab Med* 1982;**14**:55.

32 Gallon RL. Perception of disability in chronic back pain patients: a long-term follow-up. *Pain* 1989;**37**:67.

33 Deyo RA, Rainville J, Kent DL. What can the history and physical examination tell us about low back pain? *JAMA* 1992;**268**:760.

34 Deyo RA. Lumbar spine films in primary care: current use and the effects of selective ordering criteria. *J Gen Intern Med* 1986;**1**:20.

35 Deyo RA. magnetic resonance imaging of the lumbar spine: terrific test or tar baby? *N Engl J Med* 1994;**331**:115.

36 Katz JN. The assessment and management of low back pain: a critical review. *Arthritis Care Res* 1993;**6**:104–14.

37 Quebec Task Force on Spinal Disorders Report. *Spine* (Suppl), 1987.

38 Margo K. Diagnosis, treatment and prognosis in patients with low back pain. *Am Family*

Physician 1994;**49**:171–9.

39 Frymoyer JW. Back pain and sciatica. *New Engl J Med* 1988;**318**:291–300.

40 Travell J, Simons DG. *Myofascial pain and dysfunction: the trigger point manual, the lower extremities*. Baltimore: Williams and Wilkins, 1992:63–158.

41 Wolfe F, Smythe HA, Yunus MB, *et al*. The American College of Rheumatology 1990. Criteria for the classification of fibromyalgia: report of the multicenter criteria committee. *Arthritis Rheum* 1990;**33**:160–72.

42 Brown MS. The source of low back pain and sciatica. *Semin Arthritis Rheum* 1989;**18**(Suppl 2):67–72.

43 Deyo RA. Non-operative treatment of low back pain disorders: differentiating useful from useless therapy. In: Frymoyer JW, ed, *The adult spine: principles and practice*. New York: Raven, 1991:1567.

44 Deyo RA. Nonsurgical care of low back pain. *Neurosurg Clin North Am* 1991;**2**:851.

45 Loeser JD, Volinn E. Epidemiology of low back pain. *Neurosurg Clin North Am* 1991;**2**:713–8.

46 Bogduk N. Diskography. *APSJ* 1994;**3**(3):149–54.

47 Jackson RP. The facet syndrome: myth or reality? *Clin Orthop Rel Res* 1992;**279**:110–21.

48 Lewinnek GE, Warfield CA. Facet joint degeneration as a cause of low back pain. *Clin Orthop* 1986;**213**:216.

49 Selby DK, Paris SV. Anatomy of facet joints and its clinical correlation with low back pain. *Contemp Orthop* 1981;**3**:1097.

50 Giles LGF, Taylor JR. Innervation of lumbar zygapophyseal joint synovial folds. *Acta Orthop Scand* 1987;**58**:43–6.

51 Shealy CN. Facets in back and sciatic pain. A new approach to a major pain syndrome. *Minn Med* 1974;**57**:199.

52 Helbig T, Lee CK. The lumbar facet syndrome. *Spine* 1988;**13**:61.

53 Carette S, Marcoux S, Truchon R, *et al*. A controlled trial of corticosteroid injections in to facet joints for chronic low back pain. *N Engl J Med* 1991;**325**:1002.

54 Bernard TN, Cassidy JD. The sacroiliac joint syndrome. In: Frymoyer JW, ed, *The adult spine: principles and practice*. New York: Raven, 1991;2107–30.

55 Paris SV. Differential diagnosis of sacroiliac joint from lumbar spine dysfunction. In: *Proceedings of the First Interdisciplinary World Congress on Low Back Pain and its relation to the sacroiliac joint*. San Diego, 1992:313–26.

56 Daum WJ. The sacroiliac joint: an underappreciated pain generator. *Am J Orthop* 1995:475–8.

57 Schuchmann JA, Cannon CL. Sacroiliac strain syndrome: diagnosis and treatment. *Tex Med* 1986;**82**:33–6.

58 Mooney V. Understanding, examining for, and treating sacroiliac pain. *J Musculoskel Med* 1993:37–49.

59 Kanner R. *Low back pain:* 272–80.

60 Wiesel SW, Tsourmas N, Feffer HL, Citrin CM, Patronas N. A study of computer-assisted tomography I. The incidence of positive CAT scans in an asymptomatic group of patients. *Spine* 1984;**9**:549–51.

61 Boden SD, Davis DO, Dina TS, Patronas NJ, Wiesel SW. Abnormal magnetic-resonance scans of the lumbar spine in asymptomatic subjects. *J Bone Joint Surg* 1990;**72A**:403–8.

62 Anderson GBJ. The epidemiology of spinal disorders. In: Frymoyer JW, ed, *The adult spine: principles and practice*. New York: Raven, 1991:107–46.

63 Spengler DM. Degenerative stenosis of the lumbar spine. *J Bone Joint Surg* 1987;**69A**:305–8.

64 Caputy AJ, Luessenhop AJ. Long-term evaluation of decompressive surgery for degenerative lumbar stenosis. *J Neurosurg* 1992;**77**:669–76.

65 Paine KWE. Results of decompression for lumbar spinal stenosis. *Clin Orthop* 1976;**115**:96–100.

66 Hawkes CH, Roberts GM. Neurogenic and vascular claudication. *J Neurol Sci* 1978;**38**:337.

67 Kent DL, Haynor DR, Larson EB, *et al*. Diagnosis of lumbar spinal stenosis in adults: a meta-analysis of the accuracy of CT, MR, and myelography. *AJR* 1992;**158**:1135.

68 Saraste H. Long term clinical and radiological followup of spondylosis and spondylolis-

thesis. *J Ped Orthop* 1987;7:631.

69 Fredrickson BE, Baker D, Mcholick WJ, Yan HA, Lubicky JP. The natural history of spondylosis and spondylolisthesis. *J Bone Joint Surg* 1984;**66A**:699.

70 Frennered K, Danielson B, Nachemson A. Natural history of symptomatic isthmic low-grade spondylolisthesis in children and adolescents. A seven-year follow-up study. *J Pediatr Orthop* (in press.)

71 Frennered K, Danielson B, Nachemson A, Nordwall A. Mid-term follow-up of young patients fused in situ for spondylolisthesis. *Spine* 1991;14:409.

72 Seitsalo S, Osterman K, Hyvarinen H, Tallroth K, Schlenska D, Poussa M. Progression of the spondylolisthesis in children and adolescents. A long-term follow-up of 272 patients. *Spine* (in press).

73 Walker S, Cousins MJ. Failed back surgery syndrome. *Aust Fam Physician* 1994;**23**:2308–9.

74 Delamarter RB, Ross JS, Masaryk TJ, Modic MT, Bohlman HH. Diagnosis of lumbar arachnoiditis by magnetic resonance imaging. *Spine* 1990;15:304–10.

75 Loeser JC, Bigos SJ, Fordyce WE, Volinn EP. Low back pain: In: Bonica JJ, ed, *The management of pain*, 2nd edn, Pennsylvania: Lea and Febiger, 1990:1448–3.

76 North RB, Campbell JN, James CS, *et al.* Failed back surgery syndrome: five year follow-up in 102 patients undergoing repeated operation. *Neurosurgery* 1991;**28**:685–91.

77 Long DM. Failed low back syndrome. *Neurosurg Clin North Am* 1991;2:899–919.

78 Long DM, Filtzer DL, BenDebba M, Hendler NH. Clinical features of the failed-back syndrome. *J Neurosurg* 1988;**69**:61–71.

79 North RB, Campbell JN, James CS, *et al.* Failed back surgery syndrome: 5-year follow-up in 102 patients undergoing repeated operation. *Neurosurgery* 1991;**28**:685–91.

80 Gilbert TW, Kim JH, Posner JB. Epidural spinal cord compression from metastatic tumor: diagnosis and treatment. *Ann Neurol* 1978;**3**:40–51.

81 Waldvogel FA, Vasey H. Osteomyelitis: the past decade. *N Engl J Med* 1980;**303**:360.

82 Gran JT. An epidemiological survey of the signs and symptoms of ankylosing spondylitis. *Clin Rheumatol* 1985;4:161.

83 Nachemson AL. The lumbar spine: an orthopedic challenge. *Spine* 1976;1:59.

84 Liang M, Komaroff AL. Roentgenograms in primary care patients with acute low back pain: a cost-effectiveness analysis. *Arch Intern Med* 1982;**142**:1108–12.

85 Neman RI, Seres JL, Yospe LP, *et al.* Multidisciplinary treatment of chronic pain: long-term follow-up of low-back pain patients. *Pain* 1978;4:282.

86 Deyo RA, McNeish LM, Cone RO. Observer variability in the interpretation of lumbar spine radiographs. *Arthritis Rheum* 1985;**28**:1066–70.

87 Scavone JG, Latshaw RF, Rohrer GV. Use of lumbar spine films. Statistical evaluation at a university teaching hospital. *JAMA* 1981;**246**:1105–8.

88 Scavone JG, Latshaw RF, Weidner WA. Anteroposterior and lateral radiographs: an adequate lumbar spine examination. *AJR* 1981;**136**:715–7.

89 Wiessel SW, Tsourmas N, Feffer HL, Citrin CM, Patronas N. A study of computer-assisted tomography I. The incidence of positive CAT scans in an asymptomatic group of patients. *Spine* 1984:**9**:549–51.

90 Boden SD, Davis DO, Dina TS, Patronas NJ, Wiesel SW. Abnormal magnetic-resonance scans of the lumbar spine in asymptomatic subjects. A prospective investigation. *J Bone Joint Surgery* 1990;**72A**:403–8.

91 Jensen MC, Brant-Zawadski MN, Obuchowski N, *et al.* Magnetic resonance imaging of the lumbar spine in people without back pain. *N Engl J Med* 1994;**331**:69.

92 Bernard TN. Lumbar discography followed by computed tomography: refining the diagnosis of low back pain. *Spine* 1990;15:690–707.

93 Bogduk N. The lumbar disc and low back pain. *Neurosurg Clin North Am* 1991;2:791–806.

94 Bosacco N, Windsor M, Inglis A. Lumbar discography: redefining its role with intradiscal therapy. *Orthopedics* 1986;9:399–401.

95 Vanharanta H, Sachs BL, Spivey MA, *et al.* The relationship of pain provocation to lumbar disc deterioration as seen by CT/discography. *Spine* 1987;12:295–8.

96 Osti OL, Fraser RD. MRI and discography of annular tears and intervertebral disc degeneration: a prospective clinical comparison. *J Bone Joint Surg* 1992;**74B**:431–5.

97 Executive Committee of the North American Spine Society. Position statement on discography. *Spine* 1988;**13**:1343.
98 Colhoun E, McCall IW, Williams L, Cassar Pullicino VN. Provocation discography as a guide to planning operations on the spine. *J Bone Joint Surg* 1988;**70B**:267–71.
99 Nachemson A. Editorial comment: lumbar discography—where are we today? *Spine* 1989;**14**:555–7.
100 Revel ME, Listrat VM, Chevalier XJ, *et al.* Facet joint block for low back pain: identifying predictors of a good response. *Arch Phys Med Rehabil* 1992;**73**:824–8.
101 Marks RC, Houston T, Thulbourne T. Facet joint injection and facet nerve block: a randomized comparison in 86 patients with chronic low back pain. *Pain* 1992;**49**:325–8.
102 Schwarzer AC, Aprill SN, Derby R, Fortin J, Kine G, Bogduk N. The false-positive rate of uncontrolled diagnostic blocks of the lumbar zygapophysial joints. *Pain* 1994;**58**:195–200.
103 McCall I, Park WM, O'Brien JP. Induced pain referral from posterior lumbar elements in normal subjects. *Spine* 1979;**4**:441–6.
104 Mooney V, Robertson J. The facet syndrome. *Clin Orthop* 1976;**115**:149–56.
105 Eisenstein SM, Parry CR. The lumbar facet arthrosis syndrome: clinical presentation and articular surface changes. *J Bone Joint Surg* 1987;**69**:3–7.
106 Winnie AP. Differential neural blockade for the diagnosis of pain mechanisms. In: Waldman SD, Winnie AP, eds, *Interventional pain management*. Philadelphia, PA: WB Saunders, ch 12, 129–36.
107 Deyo RA, Cherkin D, Conrad D, *et al.* Cost, controversy, crisis: low back pain and the health of the public. *Ann Rev Publ Health* 1990;**12**:141.
108 Woodyard JF. Injury, compensation claims and prognosis. Part II. *J Soc Occup Med* 1980;**30**:57.
109 Spengler DM, Bigos SJ, Martin NA, Zeh J, Fisher L, Nachemson A. Back injuries in industry: a retrospective study. I. Overview and cost analysis. *Spine* 1986;**11**:241.
110 Nachemson A, Eek C, Peterson LE, Wallin L, Ohlund C, Lindstrom I. Chronic low back disability can largely be presented: a prospective randomized trial in industry. In: *AAOS 56th Annual Meeting. Las Vegas*, Feb 9–14, 1989.
111 Hoffman RM, Wheeler KJ, Deyo RA. Surgery for herniated lumbar discs: a literature synthesis. *J Gen Intern Med* 1993;**8**:487.
112 Robertson JT. The rape of the spine. *Surg Neurol* 1993;**39**:5.
113 Cassisi JE, Wypert GW, Salamon A, Kapel L. Independent evaluation of a multi-disciplinary rehabilitation program for chronic low back pain. *Neurosurgery* 1989;**25**:877–83.
114 France RD, Houpt JL, Skott A, Krishnan KRR, Varia IM. Depression as a psychopathological disorder in chronic low back pain patients. *J Psychometric Res* 1986;**30**:127–33.
115 Atkinson JH, Slater MA, Grant I, Patterson TL, Garfin SR. Depressed mood in chronic low back pain: relationship with stressful life events. *Pain* 1988;**35**:47–55.
116 Love AW. Depression in chronic low back pain patients: diagnostic efficiency of three self-report questionnaires. *J Clin Psychol* 1987;**43**:84–9.
117 Jenkins DG, Ebbutt AF, Evans CD. Tofranil in the treatment of low back pain. *J Int Med Res* 1976;**4**:41–8.
118 Gourlay GK, Cherry DA, Cousins MJ, Love BL, Graham JR, McLachlan MO. A controlled study of a serotonin reuptake blocker, zimeldine, in the treatment of chronic pain. *Pain* 1986;**25**:35–52.
119 Ward N, Bokan JA, Phillips M, Benedetti C, Butler S, Spengler D. Antidepressants in concomitant chronic back pain and depression: doxepin and desipramine compared. *J Clin Psychiatry* 1984;**45**:54–7.
120 Sullivan MJL, Reesor K, Miksail S, Fisher R. The treatment of depression in chronic low back pain: review and recommendation. *Pain* 1992;**50**:5–13.
121 Turner JA, Denny MC. Do antidepressant medications relieve chronic low back pain? *J Fam Pract* 1993;**37**:545–53.
122 Deyo RA, Diehl AK, Rosenthal M. How many days of bed rest for acute low back pain? A randomized clinical trial. *N Engl J Med* 1986;**315**:1064.
123 Koes BW, Bouter LM, Beckerman H, van der Heijden GJ, Knipschiled PG. Physiotherapy exercises and back pain: a blinded review. *BMJ* 1991;**302**:1572–6.

124 Mayer TG, Gatchel RJ, Mayer H, Kishino ND, Keeley J, Moorly V. A prospective two-year study of functional restoration in industrial low back injury. An objective assessment procedure. *JAMA* 1987;**258**:1763–7.

125 Hubbard DR, Berkoff GM. Myofascial trigger points show spontaneous needle EMG activity. *Spine* 1993;**18**:1803–7.

126 McClaflin RR. Myofascial pain syndrome: primary care strategies for early intervention. *Postgrad Med* 1994;**96**:56–73.

127 Dexter JR, Simons DS. Local twitch response in human muscle evoked by palpation and needle penetration of a trigger point. *Arch Phys Med Rehabil* 1981;**62**:521–2.

128 Kline MT. Radiofrequency techniques in clinical practice. In: Waldman, Winnie, eds, *Interventional pain management*. Philadelphia: WB Saunders, 1996: ch 17, 185–218.

129 Dilke TFW, Burry HC, Grahame R. Extradural corticosteroid injection in management of lumbar nerve root compression. *BMJ* 1973;**2**:635–7.

130 Yates DW. A comparison of the types of epidural injection commonly used in the treatment of low back pain and sciatica. *Rheumatol Rehab* 1978;**17**:181–6.

131 Racz GB, Heavner JE, Diede JH. Lysis of epidural adhesions utilizing the epidural approach. In: Waldman, Winnie, eds, *Interventional pain management*. Philadelphia: WB Saunders, 1996: ch 32, 339–52.

132 Shealy CN, Mortimer JT, Hagfors NR. Dorsal column electroanalgesia. *J Neurosurg* 1970;**32**:560–4.

133 Wester K. Dorsal column stimulation in pain treatment. *Acta Neurol Scand* 1987;**75**:151–5.

134 Marchand S, Bushnell MC, Molina-Negro P, *et al.* The effects of dorsal column stimulation on measures of clinical and experimental pain in man. *Pain* 1991;**45**:249–57.

135 Meglio M, Cioni B, Rossi GF. Spinal cord stimulation in management of chronic pain. *J Neurosurg* 1989;**70**:519–24.

136 Finch PM, Taylor JR. Functional anatomy of the spine. In: Waldman, Winnie, eds, *Interventional pain management*. Philadelphia: WB Saunders, 1996: ch 5, 39–64.

7: Cancer pain management

RICHARD B. PATT and SURESH REDDY

Introduction

Significant pain accompanies a diagnosis of cancer in about two-thirds of cases, including about 25% of patients in active treatment and up to 90% of those with advanced disease.[1] Prior to efforts of the World Health Organisation (WHO)[2] and others[3] to promote the concept of cancer pain as a major public health problem, treatment outcomes were uniformly poor,[4] or more often were not even reported. Data from more recent surveys that identify pain control as a specific outcome variable have demonstrated that 70–90% of patients will experience durable analgesia when oral medications are prescribed according to accepted guidelines.[5 6] Of the patients who fail such conservative management, most can achieve comfort with parenterally administered opioids,[7 8] especially when these techniques are combined with other more invasive approaches or procedural approaches offered by anaesthetists or neurosurgeons.[9 10] As a result, when the comprehensive cancer care is regarded as including pain and symptom control and treatment plans include pain control as a legitimate goal, it is the rare individual who should experience prolonged, intractable suffering.

Despite the encouraging nature of this preliminary outcome data, unrelieved cancer pain remains an epidemic problem, especially in less developed nations.[11] The WHO has cited three factors as being essential for maintaining effective cancer pain control at a global level: drug availability, a public health policy that sanctions appropriate drug use, and an educational programme to ensure optimal utilisation (Fig. 7.1).[12] Contemporary guidelines rely heavily on treatment with analgesics, stress cost-effective "low-tech" interventions and have been shown to be effective in up to 88% of patients.[6] Considerable effort is still required to disseminate culturally appropriate guidelines, ensure adequate drug availability and integrate contemporary practice guidelines in diverse settings where unremitting cancer pain remains all too common.

172

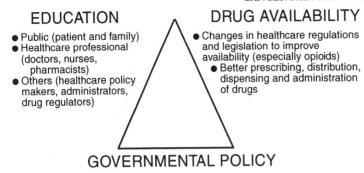

Fig 7.1   Diagrammatic representation of the three factors cited by WHO as being essential for maintaining effective cancer pain control at a global level

Assessment

Inadequate assessment is cited as one of the most common causes for undertreatment.[13] The aetiology of cancer pain can usually be determined at the bedside with the systematic application of discrete, cost-effective skills that are easily learned. While a proportion of patients will require more sophisticated diagnostic testing to confirm the aetiology of pain, these patients can usually be readily identified. Information gleaned from an initial assessment and serial re-evaluation forms the basis for therapeutic decision making, and thus adequacy of assessment is an important determinant of outcome. For example, in a study conducted at Memorial Sloan Kettering, pertinent new findings were noted by the pain service in 63% of newly evaluated patients which, in almost 20% of cases, served as the basis for instituting new antineoplastic or antibiotic therapy.[14]

The subjective and personal nature of pain requires that assessment be extended to include biological determinants (the pain syndrome, the neoplastic process, associated symptoms, intercurrent medical conditions) and psychosocial determinants (beliefs, cultural milieu, economic status, family interactions, etc.)[15] Self-report has been consistently acknowledged as the most important method of obtaining meaningful information about a person's pain.[16] While pain questionnaires have been developed and validated as a systematic means for obtaining information,[17] they are best regarded as an adjunct to a thorough history and physical examination. Although pain assessment can often be performed rapidly, it must be integrated with a more complete history and physical examination. The intensity of assessment depends in part on whether complaints are new or

173

recurring. Regardless, assessment should include surveillance for non-specific concurrent medical problems (e.g. infection, bowel obstruction, cardiopulmonary compromise), as well as problems more specific to neoplastic disease (e.g spinal cord compression, hypercalcaemia, pleural effusion).

The pain history

A pain history (Table 7.1) is obtained which, since cancer patients tend to have pain in multiple regions,[18] is initiated by eliciting an inventory of distinct pains that may be present. Detailed information is then obtained about each pain problem, starting with a history of its evolution and a description of its temporal aspects (constant, intermittent, constant with exacerbations). The patient is asked to describe the location of the pain (when possible to point to it with one finger or hand) and any areas to which it radiates. The severity of pain at best, at worst, on average and at present should be elicited. Most clinicians prefer a written or verbal 0–10 intensity scale, in which zero corresponds to an absence of pain and 10 signifies the worst pain the patient can imagine. Ultimately, the selection of a specific pain intensity scale is less important than its consistent use. Patients are asked to select the adjectives that best describe the quality of their pain either spontaneously or from a list that includes terms such as "dull, sharp, aching, gnawing, burning, tingling, shooting and pressing, etc." The presence of associated neurological or vasomotor findings such as altered sensation, motor weakness, swelling and skin changes is sought. The patient is asked to describe factors associated with increased and decreased pain, and is asked to list analgesics used presently and in the past, together with favourable and unfavourable responses.

Like a careful history, the physical examination (Table 7.2) is a relatively

Table 7.1 Elements of a comprehensive pain history

Premorbid chronic pain
Premorbid drug or alcohol use
Pain inventory (number and locations of multiple pains)
For each pain
  Onset and evolution
  Site and radiation
  Temporal pattern (constant, intermittent, predictable, etc.)
  Intensity (best, worst, average, current, 0–10 scale)
  Quality (dull, sharp, aching burning, tingling, etc.)
  Exacerbating factors (activity, position, analgesics, etc.)
  Relieving factors
  Interference with function (total pain)
  Subjective neurological and motor abnormalities
  Vasomotor changes
  Other associated factors (e.g. colour and temperature changes)
  Current analgesics (use, efficacy, side-effects)
  Prior analgesics (use, efficacy, side-effects)

Table 7.2 Components of a directed physical examination in the presence of cancer pain

---

Weight and vital signs
Auscultation of the chest
Abdominal examination
Examination of painful site and surrounding tissues
Neurological examination
Musculoskeletal examination
Examination of sites of known tumour involvement

---

non-invasive, cost-effective and time-conservative means of obtaining information.[19] Examining patients with advanced illness is challenging to the clinician and, when patients are debilitated, even a thorough examination can be demanding of their limited resources. A basic physical examination with an emphasis on neurological changes, however, is important, especially in home-bound patients whose access to routine medical care may be restricted. Although neurological and musculoskeletal findings may be difficult to interpret in the presence of acute pain, it is essential to identify simple non-oncological causes of pain (e.g. trigger points, positive straight leg raising) and signs that may suggest compression of the spinal cord and major nerve plexuses which, if present, signal the need for urgent evaluation and treatment.[20–23] Various specific pain syndromes have been recognised in cancer patients which when identified may aid in management.[1 15]

Multimodal management

Since cancer pain is often a chronic condition that typically changes over time, management is provided along a continuum, and concomitant multimodal treatment is often warranted. Treatment directed at modifying the source of pain with antineoplastic therapies is desirable, but has important limitations due to the potential for toxicity, incomplete response and latency to effect. As a result, even when antitumour therapy is instituted, treatment with analgesics is generally required to manage residual pain and to control pain while waiting for desired effects. Radiotherapy is often effective for the management of bone pain, and when the goal of treatment is palliation, can often be administered in abbreviated fractions.[24] Recently, treatment with the intravenous radioisotope strontium-89 has been shown to effectively control pain due to disseminated bone metastases in a high proportion of patients, especially with breast and prostate cancer.[25] Anaesthetic or neurosurgical interventions may be indicated for the management of refractory pain, but generally complement rather than replace relief provided by treatment with analgesics. Various non-pharmacological therapies have roles in specific settings, such as the use of psychological techniques (e.g. relaxation training, guided imagery)

Table 7.3 Favourable attributes of pharmacological therapy

Similar treatments are applicable across a wide range of ages
Similar treatments are applicable across a wide range of cultures
Similar treatments are applicable across a wide range of medical fitness
Treatment is reversible and titratable
Treatment is applicable for pain due to a variety of causes (tumour progression, treatment-related pain, premorbid chronic pain)
Treatment is effective for pain due to a variety of mechanisms (nociceptive and neuropathic)
Treatment is effective for a wide range of topographic pains (localised, multifocal, diffuse, midline pain)
Side-effects are reversible
Implementation does not depend on sophisticated technology or scarce resources

when pain is associated with anxiety, muscle tension or depression, and physical modalities, when rehabilitation is indicated.

Pharmacotherapy

Favourable attributes of pharmacological therapy are summarised in Table 7.3. With careful attention to detail, pain can usually be effectively controlled over prolonged intervals and diverse medical events with straightforward pharmacotherapy. Maintenance of pain control, however, is a time-intensive endeavour because of interindividual variability and the dynamic nature of cancer pain. WHO has adopted a "ladder" approach to cancer pain management that relies exclusively on the administration of oral agents (Fig. 7.2) and is effective in most cases. The recent introduction

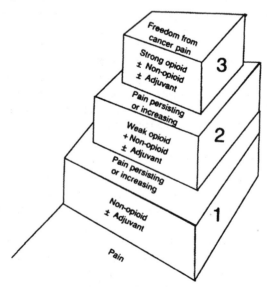

Fig 7.2 The WHO analgesic ladder (WHO, 1986)

of transdermal and oral transmucosal fentanyl provides alternative means of controlling pain non-invasively.[26-28] Pain control can be achieved in a high proportion of remaining patients when opioids are administered parenterally (subcutaneously[7] or intravenously[8]), regionally (intraspinally[9] or intraventricularly[29]), and when these techniques are combined with other more invasive approaches.[10]

Non-steroidal anti-inflammatory drugs (NSAIDs)

The NSAIDs are indicated for mild pain, and may be combined with stronger analgesics for moderate to severe pain.[30] The NSAIDs are particularly effective for pain of bony metastatic origin, as well as pain of an inflammatory nature, due to inhibitory effects on prostaglandin synthetase (cyclooxygenase),[31] an enzyme involved in prostaglandin synthesis. Regular (around-the-clock or a-t-c) administration is most effective. Gastrointestinal, haematological and renal toxicity may occur, as well as masking of fever, a particular concern in patients with reduced marrow reserves. In contrast to opioids, the use of the NSAIDs is associated with a ceiling effect, above which dose escalations do not result in enhanced analgesia. The ceiling dose in a given individual may differ from the recommended dose by up to two-fold however, and as a result some dose titration may still be indicated.[32] Selection is based on the patient's prior experience, minor differences in toxicity, physician experience, schedule, and expense.[30]

Co-analgesics/analgesic adjuvants

The so-called "adjuvant analgesics or co-analgesics" enhance opioid-mediated analgesia, reduce opioid-mediated toxicity, or help control other symptoms of cancer.[33] They are a heterogeneous group of medications developed for purposes other than relief of pain, but subsequently determined to have a complementary or occasionally primary role in pain management. For drugs with purported co-analgesic properties, evidence most strongly supports the use of selected antidepressants, anticonvulsants, oral local anaesthetics, and corticosteroids.

Co-analgesics versus opioids

In contrast to the opioids, which are relatively useful for all types of pain, the co-analgesics are indicated only in specific settings; for example, antidepressants,[33-39] anticonvulsants[33 40-42] and oral local anaesthetics[43 44] for neuropathic pain, and corticosteroids[45-49] for pain associated with inflammation and peritumoural oedema. The dose–response relationship for these drugs and the opioids differs in important ways. The administration of a sufficient dose of an opioid invariably results in some degree of analgesia, which increases linearly with the dose in a close temporal relationship to each administration. Depending on the underlying pain mechanism and other more obscure factors, administration of the co-analgesics may or may not result in analgesia. The onset of analgesia may be delayed by days or even weeks after initiating therapy, and the quality of analgesia is less closely linked to dose changes. As a result, serial trials of each class of co-analgesics, and even of different agents within the same class, may be indicated.

Opioid analgesics

The mainstay of treatment for cancer pain of moderate to severe intensity is with potent opioid analgesics, which occupy the highest tier of the three-step ladder scheme (Fig. 7.2) recommended by the WHO.[2] This treatment hierarchy can be assessed at any tier, and thus patients with severe pain may initially be prescribed potent opioids. Also of note is that when patients ascend the ladder serially, less potent analgesics should not be automatically eliminated since the NSAIDs may provide additive analgesia and the mild opioids may be useful for breakthrough or incident pain.

The various opioids produce analgesia by similar mechanisms and, when administered in comparable doses, the quality of analgesia and spectrum of side-effects are similar.[50] Nevertheless, individuals vary idiosyncratically in their sensitivity to the analgesic effects and toxicity of the various drugs (incomplete cross tolerance), forming the basis for the clinical use of morphine alternatives.[51] Other reasons for selecting alternate opioid preparations and routes include convenience of dosing and patient satisfaction, variable patterns of pain, gastrointestinal dysfunction, the need for concentrated formulations, and prior favourable clinician and patient experience.

Opioids conventionally used to treat moderate pain

Traditionally when treatment with the NSAIDs is associated with insufficient relief of pain, is contraindicated or poorly tolerated, the addition of a member of the class of drugs referred to as the "weak opioids" is recommended as an analgesic of intermediate potency.[3] Most weak opioids are available only as combination analgesics (with paracetamol (acetaminophen) or aspirin), and while there is probably no ceiling dose for the opioid component of these formulations, the number of tablets that can be taken safely is limited by their aspirin or paracetamol (acetaminophen) content. Given the lack of a ceiling dose for the opioid component of these preparations, the distinction between so-called weak and potent opioids is somewhat artificial, influenced more on a cultural rather than medical basis; for example, oxycodone has recently been made available in an uncombined form that can be utilised in progressively higher doses to treat even severe pain.[52] One of the most common prescribing errors relates to continuing the use of codeine-like drugs after they are no longer effective, in an ill-advised attempt to avoid prescribing more potent opioids which are also more highly regulated.[53]

Propoxyphene, a stereoisomer of methadone, has relatively few indications for the management of cancer pain since it is only about one-half to one-third as potent as codeine[53] and has been shown in some studies to be no more effective than aspirin or paracetamol (acetaminophen).[54] Although codeine is considered the prototypical drug of this class, its emetogenic and constipating effects are disproportionate to its relatively weak analgesic properties. Oxycodone is up to 7·7 times more potent than codeine,[55] and, of this class of drugs, is preferred by many authorities,[52] especially since it has recently been made available in a controlled release formulation that can be administered twice daily.[56] The potency of hydrocodone and dihydrocodeine lies between that of codeine and oxycodone.[57] They are typically available as combination products, and in many settings their use is preferred by clinicians because they are less highly regulated, at least in the USA.

Potent opioids: morphine

Morphine remains the standard of reference to which other analgesics are commonly compared. The pharmacokinetic and pharmacodynamic characteristics of a single 10 mg dose of morphine administered intramuscularly forms the basis of most tables and charts compiled to describe the relative characteristics of the opioids (Tables 7.4 and 7.5). Despite widespread use and extensive research, misconceptions about the use of morphine for chronic pain management continue to interfere with its optimal use (Table 7.6).[53]

Morphine is readily absorbed from the gastrointestinal tract and is metabolised in the liver. With chronic use, about one-third of the orally administered dose ultimately exerts an analgesic effect (oral bioavailability of 3:1). This is in contrast to the 6:1 parenteral:oral ratio determined from single dose studies for acute pain.[58] Since parenterally administered drug is not subject to this first-pass effect, clinicians may incorrectly perceive parenterally administered opioids as more effective than opioids administered orally. Recent research has focused on the role of morphine metabolites, once thought to be inactive. Morphine-3-glucuronide has been postulated to antagonise opioid analgesia, while morphine-6-glucuronide appears to possess potent analgesic properties and may be responsible for persistent nausea and sedation, especially in the presence of altered renal function.[59-62] The clinical relevance of these metabolites is currently uncertain.

Morphine is available in a variety of formulations and is appropriate for administration by a variety of routes. The most important distinctions are between:

179

1 So-called "immediate release preparations" which have a short latency to effect (about 30 minutes) and short duration (2–4 hours), and are usually administered every 4 or 3 hours

2 "Controlled release preparations" which have a longer latency to effect and duration, and as a result are usually administered every 12 or sometimes 8 hours.

Practical use of oral morphine

Most patients will require simultaneous treatment with two different formulations of an opioid: a long acting (basal) analgesic administered a-t-c and a short acting analgesic, administered as needed (prn). This schema is analogous to the treatment of diabetes mellitus with long acting (NPH) and short acting (regular) formulations of insulin concurrently.

Table 7.4 Comparison of pure opioid agonists commonly used in cancer pain management

Drug	Route	Equivalent dose*	Usual duration
Morphine	IM/IV/SC	10 mg	2–4 h
Immediate release morphine	Oral	30 mg†	2–4 h
Controlled release oral morphine	Oral	30 mg†	12–8 h
Morphine	Rectal	30 mg	2–4 h
Hydromorphone	IM/IV/SC	1·5 mg	2–4 h
Hydromorphone	Oral	7·5 mg	2–4 h
Hydromorphone	Rectal	7·5 mg	2–4 h
Methadone	IV	10 mg	4–12 h
Methadone	Oral	20 mg	4–12 h
Levophanol	IV	2 mg	4–8 h
Levorphanol	Oral	4 mg	4–8 h
Oxymorphone	IV	1 mg	2–6 h
Oxymorphone	Rectal	10 mg	2–6 h
Heroin	IV/IM/SC	5 mg	4–5 h
Heroin	Oral	60 mg	4–5 h
Fentanyl	IV	0·1 mg	30 min–1 h
Fentanyl	Transdermal	see Table 5.5	72 h
Oxycodone	Oral	30 mg	3–4 h
Codeine	IM/SC	130 mg	2–4 h
Codeine	Oral	200 mg	2–4 h
Hydrocodone	Oral	30 mg	2–4 h
Meperidine (pethidine)‡	Oral	300 mg	2–3 h
Meperidine (pethidine)‡	IV/IM	75 mg	3–4 h

* Dose that provides analgesia equivalent to 10 mg parenteral morphine. Cited doses are approximate, and intended to serve only as guidelines. When converting between drugs or routes, it may be advisable to reduce the new dose by 10–30% to account for interindividual variability, and titrate upwards as needed.
† Single dose studies suggest an oral:parenteral ratio of 6:1, but clinical experience with repeated doses suggests 3:1, as indicated here.
‡ Not recommended for chronic administration.
IM = intramuscular; IV = intravenous; SC = subcutaneous.

Table 7.5   Recommended dose equivalency of transdermal fentanyl*

Oral morphine (mg/day)†	Parenteral morphine (mg/day)	Transdermal fentanyl (μg/h)
45–134	8–22	25
135–224	23–37	50
225–314	38–52	75
315–404	53–67	100
405–494	68–82	125
495–584	83–97	150
585–674	98–112	175
675–764	113–127	200
765–854	128–142	225
855–944	143–157	250
945–1034	158–172	275
1035–1124	173–187	300

* Modified from manufacturer's package insert.
† This is a conservative conversion, based on a 6:1 oral:parenteral ratio for morphine, and as a result up to half of patients may require rapid upward titration.

Basal (a-t-c) analgesia

Since most oncologic pain is constant and unremitting, a time-contingent (a-t-c) schedule for the administration of analgesics is preferable to symptom-contingent (prn) administration. This strategy promotes consistent therapeutic plasma levels and avoids "roller coaster" or sine wave kinetics and dynamics characterised by alternating bouts of pain and toxicity. If analgesics are withheld until pain becomes severe, sympathetic

Table 7.6   Common misconceptions about cancer pain management and opioid therapy

Tolerance to pain relief	Patients need increasing doses of medication because they inevitably become tolerant to pain relief
Intolerance to adverse symptoms	Patients remain intolerant to adverse side-effects of analgesics
Adjuvant drugs	Relief of pain does not involve regimens of multiple classes of drugs and co-analgesics
Parenteral drugs	Severe pain calls for the administration of parenteral drugs
Addiction	Addiction is prevalent and a dangerous risk
Inevitable pain	Pain is an inevitable symptom of cancer and cannot be adequately relieved with drug treatment
Ceiling dose	There is a ceiling dose above which the opioids cannot be prescribed
Physical dependence	Patients remain physically dependent and will experience withdrawal even with gradual tapering of dose
prn administration	The opioids should be prescribed on a prn basis to manage cancer pain
Low efficacy	Cancer pain cannot be managed effectively with analgesics
Respiratory depression	Use of morphine to manage pain seriously depresses respiration and shortens life
Prognosis	Use of potent opioids to manage cancer pain implies "giving up" on the patient

arousal occurs and even potent analgesics may be ineffective. Prolonged prn administration may lead to the establishment of a pattern of anticipation and memory of pain that predisposes to persistent suffering even after a more regular administration of analgesics has been instituted.[63] Basal analgesia is usually provided by the administration of controlled release preparations of oral morphine every 12 or 8 hours, or alternatively with transdermal fentanyl, methadone, or levorphanol.

Supplemental (prn) analgesia

In addition to the above regimen, potent short acting opioids with minimal potential for accumulation (immediate release morphine, hydromorphone, oxycodone) are generally made available on an as-needed basis, usually at intervals of 2–4 hours for exacerbations of pain. Such exacerbations, referred to as breakthrough pain[64] may be spontaneous, related to specific activities (incident pain[65]) or, if the dose of the basal analgesic is insufficient, may occur regularly just prior to the next scheduled dose (end of dose failure). When incident pain has been identified, patients should be instructed to utilise rescue doses prior to activity, and in the case of end of dose failure, the dose of long acting analgesic should be raised. When frequent use of the rescue doses or escape doses is observed, the dose of basal analgesic should be increased accordingly. In such cases, relatively tolerant patients generally tolerate increments of 25–50% or more of their basal dose readily.

Initiating therapy

Since dose–response and side-effects vary widely based on a number of physiological and behavioural factors (e.g. age, previous drug history, extent of disease, etc.),[66 67] therapy should be individualised to suit the patient's needs. Effective doses often dramatically exceeded guidelines recommended in standard texts (10 mg intramuscularly, 30 mg orally), which for the most part are derived from experience with acute or postoperative pain in opioid naive patients.

Treatment with oral morphine can be started in several ways. In cases of severe pain it may be desirable to initiate therapy with parenteral morphine which can later be converted to an oral drug regimen using a 1:3 ratio. More commonly, immediate release oral morphine is administered every 3–4 hours to determine opioid requirements, following which the sum of the daily dose is halved and administered as a controlled release preparation and supplemented by rescue doses of immediate release morphine, each aliquot of which should equal 10–15% of the 24-hour dose. Alternatively, treatment can be initiated with an empirically selected dose of controlled release morphine, supplemented by appropriate doses of immediate release morphine. Regardless of the regimen that is selected, low starting doses with rapid upward titration are preferred to limit the frequency of side-effects and enhance compliance.

Dose titration

The correct dose of morphine (or a morphine-line drug) for the management of cancer pain is the dose that effectively relieves the pain without inducing intolerable side-effects. Daily doses of morphine required to adequately relieve cancer pain may vary from 60 to 3000 mg in divided doses.[5] There is no ceiling effect for morphine, i.e. an increase in the dose will always produce a concomitant increase in pain relief. The starting dose is gradually and steadily titrated upward until either pain control is achieved or side-effects occur. If dose increases result in worsening side-effects and only small increments in analgesia, the pain syndrome may be relatively opioid resistant (e.g. neuropathic pain or movement-related incident pain).[68 69] Relatively opioid-resistant pain may require alternative therapeutic approaches.

Side-effects and their management

Treatment with the opioids may be associated with side-effects although in many cases these are transient and, in most cases, manageable. Prompt identification, assessment and management of side-effects is a cornerstone to treatment. Adverse effects are often perceived of as barriers to the provision of analgesics in doses required to relieve pain effectively (dose-limiting side-effects). Most drug-related side-effects can be effectively relieved with careful management, but the same attention and skill required to tailor a pain management programme needs to be applied to selecting and titrating drugs to minimise the impact of side-effects. Patient education is essential to ensure the best outcome and to avoid confusion between manageable side-effects and allergy.[70]

A detailed account of the management of opioid side-effects is beyond the scope of this article, and is available elsewhere.[71–74] The potential for side-effects should be carefully explained and patients should be encouraged to report problems as they occur. Constipation is almost invariable and requires prophylactic and continued management with laxatives[75] on a "sliding scale" regimen that provides successively stronger laxatives until a regular bowel habit ensues.[70] The clinician should monitor for the presence of bowel obstruction and faecal impaction.

Transient nausea and sedation are relatively common when opioid therapy is initiated,[74] but with continued use, usually resolve within a few days to one week.[53 70] Patients should be reassured and encouraged to adhere to their prescribed regimen of analgesics while symptomatic treatment is instituted and, as tolerance to these effects develops, later tapered.

Reversible CNS changes associated with opioid therapy range from mild sedation to somnolence, confusion, and delirium. Mild cognitive dysfunction is relatively common but usually manageable, while severe CNS toxicity can usually be avoided. Toxicity occurs most commonly after the initiation of treatment or a dose escalation, and is usually transient.[76] Sudden cognitive changes in patients taking opioids chronically are unlikely to be related to opioid therapy, and other potential causes such as brain metastases or electrolyte disturbances should be considered.[77] Sedation is most likely to emerge as a dose-limiting side-effect in the elderly and in patients with relatively opioid-resistant pain problems (incident pain, bone metastases, nerve injury). Sedation can often be minimised by initiating opioid therapy at low doses and titrating upwards gradually. Persistent sedative effects can usually be managed by initiating symptomatic treatment with a psychostimulant (methylphenidate[33] or dextroamphetamine[78]), instituting trials of an alternate opioid or an adjuvant analgesic or consideration of an alternate therapeutic modality such as a nerve block or percutaneous cordotomy.

Other potent opioids

The pharmacokinetics and pharmacodynamics of other opioid drugs are similar to those noted for morphine, and are described in detail elsewhere.[50 53]

A formulation of transdermal fentanyl has recently been introduced which, once treatment has been established, provides relatively steady plasma levels for up to 72 hours following a single application of a 25, 50, 75 or 100 μg/h patch.[26 27] The patch's design effectively converts fentanyl to a long acting agent, although consistent, near-peak levels are not obtained for a period of 12–18 hours after the first application, and effects persist for 12–18 hours after system removal.[79] Although a useful alternative for maintaining a-t-c basal analgesia, because of its long latency to effect, transdermal fentanyl is not recommended when rapid titration is required for unstable pain.

Methadone is equipotent with morphine when administered intramuscularly, and is slightly more potent when administered orally. It possesses a long and variable half-life (13–51 hours) that may lead to drug accumulation, especially in patients who are elderly or who have renal failure. Although inexpensive, most authorities recommend its use only as a second line drug and then call for careful monitoring during the initiation of therapy and after dose increases.[80] Treatment may best be initiated by prn administration until steady state is achieved, following which the interval between a-t-c administration may vary between 4 and 12 hours. Levorphanol resembles methadone, in that due to its relatively long half-life (11 hours), accumulation may occur, dosing intervals may vary from 4 to 8 or even 12 hours, and as a result the same precautions described for methadone apply to its use.[81] A parenteral dose of 2 mg and oral dose of

184

4 mg is usually equianalgesic to 10 mg of parenteral morphine.

Hydromorphone is available in a variety of formulations and can be administered by the oral, rectal, subcutaneous and intravenous routes. It is seven to eight times more potent than morphine when administered parenterally, and enterally is about four times as potent as oral morphine (parenteral to oral dose ratio of about 5:1).[74] Administered by either route, its latency to effect and duration are relatively short (about 30 minutes and 2–4 hours respectively). The main uses of hydromorphone are for subcutaneous infusions (in view of its solubility of up to 200 mg/ml), oral breakthrough dosing, and in patients who are intolerant to morphine.

Drugs to be avoided

Pethidine/meperidine, although extensively used for postoperative pain, is not recommended for chronic administration. Its oral bioavailability is relatively low (4:1) and its duration of action is relatively short (2–3 hours). The most serious drawback to chronic administration is the potential for accumulation of norpethidine/normeperidine, a toxic metabolite with a long half-life that may cause tremors, myoclonus and seizures, especially in patients with renal failure.[82 83]

Brompton's cocktail, one of the first preparations of an oral opioid to gain clinical acceptance, is now used only infrequently. Developed at Brompton's Chest Hospital in the UK it consisted of a mixture of morphine hydrochloride (or heroin), cocaine hydrochloride, alcohol, syrup, and chloroform water. In blinded trials it has not been shown to produce analgesia that is superior to an oral opioid administered alone,[84] and its use should be discouraged because of the problems associated with titrating fixed dose combinations. Likewise, no advantage has been demonstrated for treatment with heroin,[85] although it is still sometimes used in the UK and Canada, predominantly for subcutaneous infusions by virtue of its high solubility.

Opioids with mixed agonist/antagonist activity and partial agonists are not usually recommended for the treatment of chronic cancer pain.[2 3] Differential binding to opioid receptor sites, which may confer favourable properties for acute pain management, are responsible for a relatively high incidence of psychotomimetic effects,[86] and there is usually a ceiling dose above which further dose increases are not associated with additional analgesia. Patients should not be treated concurrently with a pure agonist drug, and conversion from treatment with one class of drugs to another should be performed only cautiously because of the risk of precipitating a withdrawal reaction.

Alternate routes of administration

Between one-third and two-thirds of patients may benefit from at least the transient use of an alternate route sometime before death.[87] There is no evidence that parenteral administration produces superior analgesia to oral administration, so treatment should be reserved for conditions that render oral administration unreliable, such as weakness, dry mouth, dysphagia, nausea, vomiting, malabsorption or obstruction. Alternate routes may also be considered when an impractical number of tablets must be ingested or, acutely, when rapid induction of analgesia is required to treat a pain emergency.

Rectal administration is reliable and effective, but is usually only considered practical for short term use.[88 89] A continuous subcutaneous infusion (CSCI) or continuous intravenous infusion (CII) is usually instituted when parenteral opioids need to be administered chronically.[7 8 87 89] With adequate home care support, treatment can be initiated and maintained safely and conveniently without hospitalisation. An appropriate home infusion device should be flow calibrated, portable, battery-driven, inexpensively leased, easily taught, suitable for the addition of PCA, and equipped with alarms.

Except in selected circumstances (pre-existing indwelling catheter, severe cachexia, pain emergencies), subcutaneous administration is preferred to intravenous administration because it is easier to maintain in the home and is as reliable as intravenous administration.[89] Absorption of subcutaneously administered opioids is rapid, and steady-state plasma levels are generally approached within 1 hour.[90] Morphine and hydromorphone are most commonly employed for subcutaneous infusions, and should ideally be concentrated to permit infusion at volumes of under 1–2 ml/h in order to minimise tissue irritation. The interested reader is referred elsewhere for detailed commentary on instituting and maintaining therapy.[7 28 87 89]

Investigational routes

Morphine elixir has been successfully administered by the buccal and sublingual routes in preterminal patients for short periods of time.[91] In addition, a preparation of transmucosal fentanyl lozenge has recently been approved for the pre-emptive management of patients undergoing painful procedures, and is now in clinical trials for the treatment of cancer pain.[28] Preliminary results of treatment with opioids by these and other routes (intranasal, inhalatory, transdermal iontophoretic, vaginal, and stomal) are described elsewhere.[89]

The myth of addiction as a common outcome of medical therapy

Despite widespread use, the opioids are among the most stigmatised classes of medically available drugs. Misconceptions regarding the optimal use of opioids abound (Table 7.6), of which issues related to the potential for habituation predominate.

Tolerance, physical dependence, and psychological dependence (addiction), once considered together as part of a single syndrome, are increasingly recognised as distinct phenomena (see Table 7.7). Physical dependence and tolerance are biophysiological in nature and are almost invariably associated with chronic opioid use, and as such can be conceived of as independent and distinct from addiction. Addiction (psychological dependence)[92] is regarded as a psychologically mediated disorder with possible genetic influences that occurs only rarely as a consequence of medical use, and then idiosyncratically.[93] Given acceptance of the validity of this construct, physical dependence and tolerance need not be regarded as important impediments to the successful management of cancer pain with opioid analgesics (see discussion below). Addiction exerts only an indirect negative effect that correlates with the degree to which clinicians overestimate its risk.

Physical dependence, which also occurs with drugs other than the opioids (e.g. benzodiazepines), refers to the probability that a state of withdrawal (abstinence syndrome) will occur if drug administration is abruptly discontinued or a sufficient dose of a specific antagonist is administered. If treatment with the opioids should become unnecessary, physical dependence can be readily managed (avoided) by gradually tapering opioid doses (10–25% per day) and avoiding the use of antagonists. Tolerance exists when, over time, an increased dose of a drug is required to achieve a given effect. It is usually first manifest by a decrease in the observed duration of effect of each administered dose. When tolerance is suspected to be responsible for increased reports of pain, it can usually be countered safely and effectively by simply increasing the dose, especially since tolerance also develops to many of the adverse effects of the opioids, notably nausea and sedation.

Addiction is a complex psychobehavioural syndrome characterised by overwhelming involvement in the acquisition and non-medical use of substance despite the threat or presence of physiological and/or psychological harm.[92] Although it is a rare sequelae of medical exposure[93] and therefore should not markedly influence prescribing habits, the risk of iatrogenic addiction remains a serious concern among practitioners.[53]

Invasive and procedural approaches

Contemporary approaches to managing pain and other symptoms emphasise earlier and more liberal use of opioids, recognising their low addiction potential and overall favourable risk:benefit ratio.[94] The role of invasive pain therapies remains less well defined. Ready access to anaesthetic and neurosurgical-based interventions, however, remains an essential component of comprehensive cancer pain management, especially for the 10–30% of patients whose pain remains refractory to traditional analgesic therapies.

Table 7.7 *Contemporary* description of phenomena *historically* associated with addiction

Phenomena	Aetiology	Definition	Incidence	Management
Physical dependence	Physiological, pharmacological	Withdrawal if opioids are abruptly stopped or naloxone is administered	Almost invariable	Gradual taper
Tolerance*†	Physiological, pharmacological	Increased dose required to achieve analgesia	Almost invariable	Re-establish analgesia with upward titration
Addiction (psychological dependence)	Psychobehavioural, possible genetic influences	Compulsive non-medical use despite harm	Rare (<1%)	Identify, multidisciplinary management
Withdrawal (abstinence syndrome)	Physiological, pharmacological	Characteristic signs and symptoms‡	Almost invariable	Avoid, reverse with opioids

* Incidence and severity of tolerance is now believed not to be as great as once thought; need for dose increases in cancer patients more commonly reflects disease progression.

† Tolerance develops to most adverse effects as well, especially nausea and sedation, but slowly if at all to constipation.

‡ Characteristic signs and symptoms include lacrimation, diaphoresis, rhinorrhoea, pupillary dilatation, gooseflesh, muscle tremor, nausa and vomiting, abdominal cramping, diarrhoea, raised heart rate, respiratory rate and blood pressure, chills, hyperthermia, flushing, yawning, restlessness, irritability, anorexia, disturbed sleep, and generalised body aches.

Table 7.8   Interventional approaches for controlling cancer pain

Procedure	Usual indication	Examples
Local anaesthetic blocks with or without corticosteroids	Diagnostic blocks Prognostic blocks Acute pain, muscle spasm Premorbid chronic pain Postsurgical syndromes Herpes zoster	Stellate ganglion Coeliac plexus block Trigger point injection Epidural steroids Intercostal block Subcutaneous infiltration
Neurolytic (neuroblative) blocks	Localised refractory pain that is expected to persist, usually in the presence of	Alcohol coeliac plexus block Phenol intercostal block
Ablative neurosurgery	short life expectancy, and localised to a region where treatment is associated with a low risk of neurological morbidity	Percutaneous cordotomy Midline myelotomy
Neuroaugmentative (spinal) analgesics	Refractory pain, usually in lower body, but may be widespread or diffuse	Externalised epidural catheter, intrathecal catheter with port or implanted pump

A variety of alternatives to systemic analgesics has been advocated for controlling cancer pain (Table 7.8). These approaches are generally reserved for pain that is refractory to traditional pharmacotherapies because they tend to be associated with greater acute risk, maintenance may be more demanding of institutional and family resources, and specialised skills are required for their implementation.[95 96] A small subset of these treatments may be considered relatively early in specific settings (Table 7.9).[97]

Anaesthetic and neurosurgical approaches to managing cancer pain are fundamentally of two types (Table 7.8). Neuroablation or chemical neurolysis involves intentionally injuring the nervous structures implicated in the transmission of pain. Needles are usually inserted percutaneously under radiological guidance to facilitate the injection of ethyl alcohol or phenol and, less frequently, specialised equipment is used to heat or freeze needle tips to induce more localised nerve injury. The second common

Table 7.9   Early consideration of neurolysis*

Procedure	Indication
Coeliac plexus neurolysis	Abdominal pain, back pain
Superior hypogastric plexus neurolysis	Pelvic pain
Phenol saddle block	Perineal pain with urinary diversion
Thoracic subarachnoid neurolysis	Focal chest wall pain
Intercostal neurolysis	Focal chest wall pain
Lumbar subarachnoid neurolysis	Unilateral leg pain in bed bound patient

* The risk:benefit ratio of these procedures in the specified settings is sufficiently favourable and well established to warrant early consideration.

anaesthetic/neurosurgical approach to managing cancer pain involves the placement of a catheter in the epidural or subarachnoid space for the infusion of opioids, local anaesthetics and other analgesics. Electrical stimulation, which may be employed transcutaneously (TENS), at the level of the epidural space and even to deep brain structures is mostly pertinent to the management of chronic non-malignant pain, and is infrequently employed in clinical practice for cancer pain.

Local anaesthetic blocks

Because their effect is typically transient, local anaesthetic blocks play a relatively limited role in the management of well-established cancer pain.[98] Local anaesthetic neural blockade may be performed for diagnostic, prognostic or therapeutic purposes. Diagnostic and prognostic nerve blocks help characterise the underlying mechanism of pain (somatic, visceral, sympathetic, neuropathic), and may be predictive of the potential for a subsequent neurolytic block to relieve pain or produce side-effects.

Local anaesthetic injections with or without the addition of corticosteroids may provide lasting relief in specific settings such as muscle spasm, postsurgical nerve impingement, herpes zoster, sympathetic dystrophy and premorbid chronic low back pain. Therapeutic local anaesthetic injections are associated with relatively low risks, can often be performed at the bedside and, under selected circumstances, may be rendered by a non-anaesthetist.

Neuroablative and neurolytic procedures

Neurolytic blocks have a limited but important role in the management of refractory cancer pain, especially when pain is well localised or associated with movement.[97] Treatment is usually reserved for pain that is severe and expected to persist, and is usually reserved for patients with a limited life expectancy. While complications due to needle placement and aberrant spread of neurolytic solutions may be quite serious, they are infrequent when these techniques are employed by experienced personnel with access to radiological guidance.[96] The most important factors limiting more widespread application are the potential for the development of new neuropathic pain that may arise after the block has worn off, and the risk of muscle paresis when mixed sensorimotor nerves are targeted. Well-controlled studies of neurolysis are lacking, but large clinical series report significant relief of pain in 50–80% of patients, with the best results obtained in patients who have received multiple blocks.[99 100]

Specific nerve block procedures

Peripheral neurolysis

Technically a nerve block can be performed at almost any site. Blockade of peripheral nerves has the greatest potential for producing new pain due to neuritis or deafferentiation, and because most peripheral nerves subserve both sensory and motor function, peripheral neurolysis is reserved for limited indications.[101] Pain due to rib fracture or metastasis may respond favourably to intercostal block, which is a relatively straightforward procedure that rarely results in pneumothorax. In addition, cranial nerves V and, more rarely, IX and X, and their branches, are occasionally blocked for well-localised head and neck pain. These latter procedures are more technically demanding and require fluoroscopic or CT guidance. Neurolysis of peripheral nerves subserving limb function (e.g. brachial plexus) are avoided except in imminently preterminal patients or when the limb is already rendered useless by tumour invasion.

Subarachnoid neurolysis

Subarachnoid injections of alcohol and phenol require considerable skill and specialised training and must be performed carefully to avoid unwanted neurological deficit. They may, however, be extremely useful for the management of chest wall pain and for perineal pain in patients with urinary diversions.[99 100] Discrete areas of analgesia can be obtained when small volumes are injected and the patient is positioned carefully to restrict the spread of the injected alcohol or phenol which are hypo- and hyperbaric, respectively, compared with CSF. These procedures can usually be performed on an outpatient basis without radiological guidance or special equipment and are suitable for aged or debilitated patients. Subarachnoid neurolysis frequently needs to be repeated in order to obtain durable analgesia without unwarranted risks of undesired neurological sequelae.

Sympathetic nerve blocks

Sympathetic nerve blocks are often considered relatively early since the appearance of neuritis or new pain is rare.[97 102] In addition, because fibres innervate vascular and viscera and do not subserve somatic motor or sensory function, neurological deficit is unlikely. Coeliac plexus block (Fig. 7.3) is one of the most efficacious and common nerve blocks used to provide prolonged relief of cancer pain. It is indicated for upper abdominal and back pain secondary to malignant neoplasms of the pancreas, stomach, liver and other abdominal viscera. A variety of approaches (e.g. posterior, anterior, transaortic, intraoperative) have been advocated, most of which require fluoroscopic or CT guidance because of the plexus' proximity to the abdominal aorta and other vital structures. Complication rates are uniformly low and favourable results are reported in 70–90% of patients in large series.[102] Superior hypogastric plexus block[97] is likewise very effective for pelvic pain, and is associated with minimal risks of bladder or limb paresis.

191

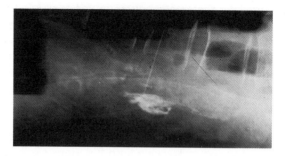

Fig 7.3   Coeliac plexus block

Intraspinal analgesia

Spinal drug therapy involves administering relatively small quantities of drugs in the epidural or intrathecal space near their receptors to enhance analgesia and, by limiting dose, to reduce adverse effects.[103] Treatment usually involves the continuous administration of opioids, the effects of which are predominantly mediated by the substantia gelatinosa of the spinal cord's dorsal horn. As opposed to spinal anaesthesia, spinal opioid analgesia is highly selective, in that pain relief occurs in the absence of changes in motor, sympathetic and sensory function. Dilute local anaesthetics may need to be added in patients with refractory pain, especially pain that is associated with movement or nerve injury, but this can often be accomplished with low concentrations that preserve motor power. Some of the favourable characteristics of spinal analgesia are that it is non-destructive, reversible, can be titrated to effect, and simple, cost-effective screening usually identifies appropriate candidates. Whilst it is most commonly considered for lower extremity and truncal pain, treatment can often be extended for disseminated and more widespread pain. Side-effects such as respiratory depression, nausea and vomiting, pruritus, urinary retention, and dysphoria can be problematical in opioid naive patients, but they are infrequent in those who have been exposed to morphine chronically.

Maintenance of spinal analgesia ultimately depends on establishing reliable access to the intrathecal or epidural space. An intraventricular approach[103] is infrequently used, and then primarily for intractable head and neck pain. The institution of spinal therapy thus requires the participation of an anaesthetist or neurosurgeon familiar with techniques of screening, implantation and maintenance, as well as a reliable home environment and nursing care. A standard epidural catheter can be taped to the back and used for short intervals to manage acute pain or pain in preterminal patients, while minor surgery is required to implant more durable drug delivery systems. A modified Hickman/Broviac catheter is usually tunnelled, externalised and attached to an ambulatory pump for treatment expected to persist for several months, and a fully implanted infusion pump is usually considered for longer durations of therapy. Despite a high initial cost, the latter system becomes cost effective over time, can be programmed with a lap top computer, and is less likely to become infected or to migrate than externalised systems.[103]

Neurosurgical approaches

Neuroablative surgery

Although ready access to neurosurgical opinion and intervention is an important component of a comprehensive cancer pain control programme, only a few procedures are performed today with any frequency. The spectrum of analgesic neurosurgical operations has been extensively reviewed elsewhere.[104] The procedure in main use is percutaneous cordotomy,[104 105] which is especially well suited for unilateral pain confined to the trunk or lower limb. It involves the percutaneous insertion of a probe beneath the mastoid process between the C1 and C2 vertebrae, and localisation of its tip within the lateral spinothalamic tract of the spinal cord. Cordotomy is ideally suited for the treatment of intractable unilateral lower extremity pain because preservation of proprioception, tactile sensation and motor strength result in a minimum of dysfunction. When more extensive lesioning is performed to produce higher levels of analgesia, or cordotomy is carried out in patients with pulmonary dysfunction, the incidence of both inadequate pain relief and complications increases. Of greatest concern is the risk of Ondine's curse, a sleep apnoea syndrome that, once established, has a high rate of mortality.

Neuromodulation

Spinal drug delivery systems may be placed and maintained by either a neurosurgical or anaesthesia team. Spinal cord stimulation, which is increasingly being advocated for chronic pain of non-malignant origin, is rarely considered appropriate for the treatment of cancer pain.

Conclusion

The prospect of suffering from unrelieved pain is one of the most feared aspects of a cancer diagnosis for most patients and their families, yet has only recently become an important focus of comprehensive cancer care. Comprehensive management involves careful assessment, individualisation of therapy, close follow-up, and a proactive approach to treatment. Adequate control of pain can be achieved in the vast majority of patients with a rigorous and aggressive application of measures that are ultimately straightforward. Anaesthetic procedures comprise an important category of complementary therapies that, when carefully selected, promote improved outcome.

References

1 Portenoy RK. Cancer pain: epidemiology and syndromes. *Cancer* 1989;**63**:2307.
2 World Health Organisation. *Cancer pain relief.* Geneva: World Health Organisation, 1986.
3 American Pain Society. *Principles of analgesic use in the treatment of acute pain and chronic cancer pain*, 3rd edn. Skokie, IL: American Pain Society, 1992.
4 Bonica JJ, Ekstrom JL. Systemic opioids for the management of cancer pain: an updated review. *Adv Pain Res Ther* 1990;**14**:425–6.
5 Ventafridda V, Tambutini M, Carceni A, *et al.* A validation study of the WHO method for cancer pain relief. *Cancer* 1987;**59**:850.
6 Zech DFJ, Grond J, Lynch J, Hertel D, Lehmann KA. Validation of World Health Organisation guidelines for cancer pain relief: a 10 year prospective study. *Pain* 1995;**63**:65–76.
7 Bruera E, Brenneis C, Macmillan K *et al.* The use of the subcutaneous route for the administration of narcotics. *Cancer* 1988;**62**:407–11.
8 Portenoy RK, Moulin DE, Rogers A, *et al.* IV infusion of opioids for cancer pain: clinical review and guidelines for use. *Cancer Treat Rep* 1986;**70**:575–81.
9 Ventafridda V, Spoldi E, Caraceni A, *et al.* Intraspinal morphine for cancer pain. *Acta Anaesthesiol Scand* 1987;**31**:(suppl 85):47.
10 Patt RB, Jain S. Therapeutic decision making for invasive procedures. In: Patt RB, ed., *Cancer pain.* Philadelphia: JB Lippincott, 1993:275–84.
11 Swerdlow M, Stjernsward J. Cancer pain relief: an urgent problem. *World Health Forum* 1982;**3**:325–30.
12 Macdonald N. Educational programs in pain and palliative care. *J Pain Symptom Management* 1993;**8**:348–52.
13 VonRoenn JH, Cleeland CS, Gronin R, *et al.* Physician attitudes and practice in cancer pain management: A survey from the Eastern Cooperative Oncology Group. *Ann Intern Med* 1993;**119**:121–6.
14 Gonzales GR, Elliot KJ, Portenoy RK, *et al.* The impact of a comprehensive evaluation in the management of cancer pain. *Pain* 1991;**47**:141–4.
15 Patt RB. Classification of cancer pain and cancer pain syndromes. In: Patt RB, ed, *Cancer pain.* Philadelphia: JB Lippincott: 3–39.
16 Grossman SA, Sheidler VR, Sweeden K, *et al.* Correlation of patient and caregiver ratings of cancer pain. *J Pain Symptom Management* 1991;**6**:53.
17 Daut RL, Cleeland CS, Flanery RC. Development of the Wisconsin brief pain questionnaire to assess pain in cancer and other diseases. *Pain* 1983;**17**:197.
18 Twycross RG. Incidence of pain. *Clin Oncol* 1984;**3**:5.
19 Longmire D. The physical examination: methods and application in the clinical evaluation of pain. *Pain Digest* 1991;**1**:136–43.
20 Jaeckle KA, Young DF, Foley KM. The natural history of lumbosacral plexopathy in cancer. *Neurology* 1985;**35**:8–15.
21 Gilbert RW, Kim JH, Posner JB. Epidural spinal cord compression from metastatic tumor: diagnosis and treatment. *Ann Neurol* 1978;**3**:40–51.
22 Kori SH, Foley KM, Posner JB. Brachial plexus lesions in patients with cancer: 100 cases. *Neurology* 1981;**31**:45.
23 Smith JL. Oncologic emergencies. In: Patt RB, ed, *Cancer pain.* Philadelphia: JB Lippincott, 1993:527–41.
24 Ashby M. Palliative radiotherapy. In: Patt RB, ed, *Cancer pain.* Philadelphia: JB Lippincott, 1993:235–50.
25 Campa J. Strontium-89: a new therapeutic alternative for bone pain of malignant origin. *Am Pain Soc Bull* 1994; Jan–Feb 6–8.
26 Ahmedzai S, Allan E, Fallon M, *et al.* Transdermal fentanyl in cancer pain. *J Drug Dev* 1994;**6**:93–7.
27 Yee LY, Lopez JR. Transdermal fentanyl. *Ann Pharmacother* 1992;**26**:1393–9.
28 Fine PG, Marcus M, De Boer AJ, Van der Oord B. An open label study of oral transmucosal fentanyl citrate for the treatment of breakthrough cancer pain. *Pain* 1991;**45**:149–53.

29 Roquefeuil B, Benezech J, Blanchet P, *et al.* Intraventricular administration of morphine in patients with neoplastic intractable pain. *Surg Neurol* 1984;21:155–8.

30 Stambaugh J. Role of nonsteroidal anti-inflammatory drugs. In: Patt RB, ed, *Cancer pain.* Philadelphia: JB Lippincott, 1993:105–18.

31 Galasko CSB. *Skeletal metastases.* London: Butterworths, 1986:99–124.

32 Portenoy R. Drug therapy for cancer pain. *Am J Hospice Pall Care* 1990;7:10.

33 Bruera E, Ripamonti C. Adjuvants to opioid analgesics. In: Patt RB, ed. *Cancer pain.* Philadelphia: JB Lippincott, 1993:185–94.

34 Watson C, Evans R, Reed K, *et al.* Amitriptyline versus placebo in post-herpetic neuralgia. *Neurology* 1982;32:671–3.

35 Kishore-Kumar R, Max MB, Schafer SC, *et al.* Desipramine relieves post-herpetic neuralgia. *Clin Pharmacol Ther* 1990;47:305–72.

36 Panerai AE, Monza G, Mouilia P, *et al.* A randomized, within-patient, crossover, placebo-controlled trial on the efficacy and tolerability of the tricyclic antidepressants chlorimipramine and nortriptyline in central pain. *Acta Neurol Scand* 1990;82:34–8.

37 Sindrup SH, Ejlertsen B, Froland A, *et al.* Imipramine treatment in diabetic neuropathy: relief of subjective symptoms without changes in peripheral and autonomic nerve function. *Eur J Clin Pharmacol* 1989;37:151–3.

38 Sindrup SH, Gram LF, Skjold T, *et al.* Clomipramine vs desipramine vs placebo in the treatment of diabetic neuropathy symptoms: a double-blind cross-over study. *Br J Clin Pharmacol* 1990;30:683–91.

39 Walsh TD. Controlled study of imipramine and morphine in chronic pain due to cancer. *Proc Am Soc Clin Oncol* 1986;5:237.

40 Swerdlow M. The use of anticonvulsants in the management of cancer pain. In: Erdmann W, Oyamma T, Pernak MJ, eds. *The pain clinic.* Utrecht, Netherlands: VNU Science Press, 1985.

41 Sweet WH. Treatment of trigeminal neuralgia (tic douloureux). *N Engl J Med* 1986;315:174–7.

42 Hatangdi VS, Boas RA, Richard EG. Postherpetic neuralgia: management with antiepileptic and tricyclic drugs. *Adv Pain Res Ther* 1976;1:583–7.

43 Dejgard A, Petersen P, Kastrup J. Mexiletine for treatment of chronic painful diabetic neuropathy. *Lancet* 1988;i:9–11.

44 Lindstrom P, Lindblom U. The analgesic effect of tocainide in trigeminal neuralgia. *Pain* 1987;28:45–50.

45 Shell H. Adrenal corticosteroid therapy in far-advanced cancer. *Geriatrics* 1972;27:131–41.

46 Moertel C, Shutte A, Reitemeir R, *et al.* Corticosteroid therapy in pre-terminal gastrointestinal cancer. *Cancer* 1974;33:1607–9.

47 Bruera E, Roca E, Cedaro L, *et al.* Action of oral methylprednisolone in terminal cancer patients: a prospective randomized double-blind study. *Cancer Treat Rep* 1985;69:751–4.

48 Della Luna GR, Pellegrini A, Piazzi M. Effects of methylprednisolone sodium succinate on quality of life in preterminal cancer patients: a placebo-controlled, multicenter study. *Eur J Cancer Clin Oncol* 1989;25:1817–21.

49 Popiela T, Lucchi R, Giongo F. Methylprednisolone as palliative therapy for female terminal cancer patients. *Eur J Cancer Clin Oncol* 1989;25:1823–9.

50 Jaffe JH. Drug addiction and drug abuse. In: Gilman AG, Goodman LS, Rall TW, *et al*, eds, *The pharmacological basis of therapeutics,* 7th edn. New York: Macmillan, 1985:532.

51 Galer BS, Coyle N, Pasternak GW, Portenoy RK. Individual variability in the response to different opioids: report of five cases. *Pain* 1992;49:87–91.

52 Kalso E, Vainio A. Morphine and oxycodone hydrochloride in the management of cancer pain. *Clin Pharm Ther* 1990;47:639–46.

53 Hill CS. Oral opioid analgesics. In: Patt RB, ed, *Cancer pain.* Philadelphia: JB Lippincott, 1993:129–42.

54 Cooper SA, Beaver WT. A model to evaluate mild analgesics in oral surgery patients. *Clin Pharmacol Ther* 1976;20:241.

55 Sunshine A, Laska EM, Olson NZ. Analgesic effects of oral oxycodone and codeine in the treatment of patients with postoperative, postfracture, or somatic pain. *Adv Pain Res Ther* 1986;8:225.

56 Kaiko R, Benziger DP, Ditzmartin RD, *et al.* Pharmacokinetic/pharmacodynamic relationships of controlled-release oxycodone. *Clin Pharmacol Ther* 1996;59:52–61.

57 Hopkinson III JH. Vicodin: a new analgesic: clinical evaluation of efficacy and safety of repeated doses. *Curr Ther Res* 1978;24:633–45.

58 Kaiko RF. Commentary: equianalgesic dose ratio of intramuscular/oral morphine, 1:6 vs 1:3. *Adv Pain Res Ther* 1986;8:87–93.

59 Portenoy RK, Foley KM, Stulman J, *et al.* Plasma morphine and morphine-6-glucuronide during chronic morphine therapy for cancer pain: plasma profiles, steady-state concentrations and the consequences of renal failure. *Pain* 1991;47:13–9.

60 Portenoy RK, Thaler HT, Inturrisi CE, Friedlander M, Foley KM. The metabolite morphine-6-glucuronide contributes to the analgesia produced by morphine infusion in patients with pain and normal renal function. *Clin Pharmacol Ther* 1992;51:422–31.

61 Sawe J. Morphine and its 3- and 6-glucuronides in plasma and urine during chronic administration in cancer patients. *Adv Pain Res Ther* 1986;5:45.

62 Smith MT, Watt JA, Cramond T. Morphine-3-glucuronide: a potent antagonist of morphine analgesia. *Life Sci* 1990;47:579.

63 Paalzow LK. Pharmacokinetic aspects of optimal pain treatment. *Acta Anaesthesiol Scand Suppl* 1982;74:37–43.

64 Portenoy RK. Breakthrough pain: definition and management. *Oncology* 1983;3:25–9.

65 Rogers AG. How to manage incident pain. *J Pain Symptom Management* 1987;2:99.

66 Kaiko RF, Wallenstein SL, Rogers AG, *et al.* Sources of variation in analgesic responses in cancer patients with chronic pain receiving morphine. *Pain* 1983;15:191–200.

67 Cleeland CS, Tearnan BH. Behavioral control of cancer pain. In: Holzman AD, Turk DC, eds, *Pain management.* New York: Pergamon, 1986:193–212.

68 Portenoy RK, Foley KM, Inturrisi CE. The nature of opioid responsiveness and its implications for neuropathic pain: new hypotheses derived from studies of opioid infusions. *Pain* 1990;43:273–86.

69 McQuay HJ. Pharmacological treatment of neuralgic and neuropathic pain. *Cancer Surv* 1988;7:29.

70 Ellison NM. Opioid analgesics: toxicities and their treatment. In: Patt RB, ed, *Cancer pain.* Philadelphia: JB Lippincott, 1993:185–94.

71 Cummings-Ajemian I. Treatment of related symptoms. In: Patt RB, ed, *Cancer pain.* Philadelphia: JB Lippincott, 1993:197–208.

72 Smith JL. Care of people who are dying: the hospice approach. In: Patt Rb, ed, *Cancer pain.* Philadelphia: JB Lippincott, 1993: 543–52.

73 Baines M. Nausea and vomiting in the patient with advanced cancer. *J Pain Symptom Management* 1988;3:81–5.

74 Levy MH. Pain management in advanced cancer. *Semin Oncol* 1985;12:394.

75 Twycross RG, Harcourt JMV. The use of laxatives at a palliative care center. *Palliative Med* 1991;5:27.

76 Bruera E, MacMillan K, Hanson J. The cognitive effects of the administration of narcotic analgesics in patients with cancer pain. *Pain* 1989;39:13–6.

77 Bruera E, Chadwick S, Winlick A, *et al.* Delirium and severe sedation in a patient with terminal cancer. *Cancer Treat Rep* 1987;71:787.

78 Forrest W, Brown B, Brown C, *et al.* Dextro-amphetamine with morphine for the treatment of postoperative pain. *N Engl J Med* 1977;296:712.

79 Portenoy RK, Southam MA, Gupta SK, *et al.* Transdermal fentanyl for cancer pain: repeated dose pharmacokinetics. *Anesthesiology* 1993;78:36–43.

80 Ettinger DS, Vitale PJ, Trump DL. Important clinical pharmacologic considerations in the use of methadone in cancer patients. *Cancer Treat Rep* 1979;63:457.

81 Dixon R. Pharmacokinetics of levorphanol. *Adv Pain Res Ther* 1986;8:217.

82 Kaiko RF, Foley KM, Grabinski PY, *et al.* Central nervous system excitatory effects of meperidine in cancer patients. *Ann Neurol* 1983;13:180–5.

83 Inturrisi CE, Umans JG. Meperidine biotransformation and central nervous system toxicity in animals and humans. *Adv Pain Res Ther* 1986;8:143.

84 Melzack R, Mount BM, Gordon JM. The Brompton mixture vs morphine solution given orally: effects on pain. *Can Med Assoc J* 1979;120:435–8.

85 Twycross RG. The measurement of pain in terminal carcinoma. *J Int Med Res*

1976;4:58–67.

86 Martin WR. Pharmacology of opioids. *Pharmacol Rev* 1984;35:283.

87 Coyle N, Adelhardt J, Foley KM, Portenoy RK. Character of terminal illness in the advanced cancer patient: pain and other symptoms during the last four weeks of life. *J Pain Symptom Management* 1990;5:83–93.

88 Cole L, Hanning CD. Review of the rectal use of opioids. *J Pain Symptom Management* 1990;5:118–26.

89 Bruera E, Ripamonti C. Alternate routes of administration of narcotics. In: Patt RB, ed, *Cancer pain*. Philadelphia: JB Lippincott, 1993:161.

90 Nahata MC, Miser AW, Miser JS, *et al*. Analgesic plasma concentrations of morphine in children with terminal malignancy receiving a continuous subcutaneous infusion of morphine sulfate to control severe pain. *Pain* 1987;18:109–14.

91 Enck RE. Mucosal membranes as alternative routes for morphine sulfate administration. *Am J Hospice Care* 1988;11:17–8.

92 Rinaldi RC, Steindler EM, Wilford BB, *et al*. Clarification and standardization of substance abuse terminology. *JAMA* 1988;259:555.

93 Porter J, Jick H. Addiction rate in patients treated with narcotics. *N Engl J Med* 1980;302:123.

94 Jacox A, Carr DB, Payne R, *et al*. Management of cancer pain: clinical practice guidelines No 9. Rockville, MD: AHCPR Publication No. 94-0592; March 1994.

95 Patt RB, Jain S. Therapeutic decision making for procedure-based pain. In: Patt RB, ed, *Cancer pain*, 1993:275–83.

96 Jain S, Patt RB. Complications of invasive procedures. In: Patt RB, ed, *Cancer pain*, 1993:443–60.

97 Patt RB, Jain S, *et al*. The outcomes movement and neurolytic blockade for cancer pain management. *Pain Digest* 1995;5:268–77.

98 Abrams SE. The role of non-neurolytic blocks in the management of cancer pain. In: Abrams SE, ed, *Cancer pain*. Boston; Kluwer Academic, 1989:67–75.

99 Hay RC. Subarachnoid alcohol block in the control of intractable pain: report of results in 252 patients. *Anesth Analg* 1962;41:12–6.

100 Papo I, Visca A. Phenol subarachnoid rhizotomy for the treatment of cancer pain: a personal account of 290 cases. *Adv Pain Res Ther* 1979;2:339–46.

101 Patt RB. Peripheral neurolysis and the management of cancer pain. *Pain Digest* 1992;2:30–42.

102 Eisenberg E, Carr, DB, Chalmers TC. Neurolytic celiac plexus block for treatment of cancer pain: a meta-analysis. *Anesth Analg* 1995;80:290–5.

103 Waldman S, Leak D, Kennedy D, Patt RB. Intraspinal opioid analgesia in the management of oncologic pain. In: Patt RB, ed, *Cancer pain*. Philadelphia: JB Lippincott, 1993:285–328.

104 White JC, Sweet WH. *Pain and the neurosurgeon: a forty year experience*. Springfield, IL: Charles C Thomas, 1969.

105 Patt RB. Pain therapy. In: Frost EAM, ed, *Clinical anesthesia in neurosurgery*, 2nd edn, Boston: Butterworths, 1990.

8: Interventional techniques

PRITHVI RAJ

In patients with persisiting intolerable pain lasting for longer than 3 months, it is necessary to find new avenues of pain management. Prolonged analgesia is one of those techniques which is indicated in such patients. This can be provided by performing special procedures such as epidural analgesia with PCA, implantable drug-delivery systems, spinal cord and peripheral nerve stimulation, radiofrequency and cryolysis. Epidural analgesia is described in Chapter 3. Description of the other techniques follow.

Implantable drug-delivery systems

Intraspinal narcotics have dramatically influenced the way pain of malignant origin is managed; this is seen by the continued decline in the number of neurodestructive procedures performed to palliate cancer pain.[1] This powerful modality has been expanded to treat selected patients suffering from chronic benign pain.[2] In tandem, various implantable drug-delivery systems have been developed to complement and facilitate the delivery of opioids and other drugs to the neuraxis.

Classification

Table 8.1 describes the six basic types of implantable drug-delivery systems. The Type I system, a simple percutaneous catheter analogous to

Table 8.1   Spinal drug delivery systems

Type I	Percutaneous epidural or subarachnoid catheter
Type II	Percutaneous epidural or subarachnoid catheter with subcutaneous tunnelling
Type III	Totally implanted epidural or subarachnoid catheter with subcutaneous injection port
Type IV	Totally implanted epidural or subarachnoid catheter with implanted manually activated pump
Type V	Totally implanted epidural or subarachnoid catheter wtih implanted infusion pump
Type VI	Totally implanted epidural or subarachnoid catheter with implanted programmable infusion pump

those used for obstetric pain control, is the type that anaesthetists are most familiar with. The Type II system is simply a catheter suitable for percutaneous placement and tunnelling. The Type III system consists of a totally implantable injection port that is attached to a Type II tunnelled catheter. The Type IV system is a totally implantable, mechanically activated pump attached to a Type II tunnelled catheter and is, in principle, a PCA device. The Type V system is a totally implantable continuous infusion pump that is connected to a Type II tunnelled catheter. The Type VI system is a totally implantable programmable infusion pump attached to a Type II tunnelled catheter. The programmable feature of the Type VI implantable drug-delivery system allows a broad spectrum of delivery rates and modes, including occasional bolus injections.

Each of these drug-delivery systems has a unique profile of advantages and disadvantages.[3] The pain management specialist must be familiar with the particular merits of each system if optimal selection is to be made. In this time of increasing pressure to control the costs of health care, economic factors must also play a role in the selection of an implantable drug-delivery system. The cost of both the intended delivery system and the drugs to be administered through the delivery system must be considered prior to implantation of an implantable drug-delivery system. A perfectly functioning implantable drug-delivery system is of no value to the patient who is unable to pay for the drugs, special needles, and supplies needed to use the delivery system. Similarly, implanted systems may superimpose financial hardship upon a difficult terminal course. With prior planning, the financial issues can be individualised and resolved.

Issues to be considered prior to device placement

Appropriate patient selection is crucial if optimal results are to be achieved, in terms of pain palliation and patient satisfaction. Factors that must be considered prior to placement of an implantable drug-delivery system are summarised in Table 8.2.[12] These issues will be discussed further.

Table 8.2   Preimplantation considerations

Result of preimplantation trials of spinal drugs
Infection
Clotting disorders
Behavioural abnormalities
Physiological abnormalities
Cost of delivery system
Cost of drugs, needles and supplies
Evaluation of support system
Concurrent therapy
Life expectancy

Preimplantation trial

The first responsibility to the patient being considered for an implantable drug-delivery system is to make a diagnosis of the pain problem and analyse the appropriateness of the patient's current analgesic regimen. A pre-implantation trial of spinal opioids is necessary to determine whether an implantable drug-delivery system can adequately relieve the patient's pain. Not all pain is relieved by spinal opioids.[4] An implantable drug-delivery system should never be implanted without first verifying the ability of the spinal drug being considered to relieve the patient's symptoms adequately on two separate occasions. Extensive clinical experience suggests that implantation should not proceed unless the magnitude of relief is less than 50% of the preinjection intensity, with a duration of at least twice the half-life of the agent; for example, 8–12 hours in the case of morphine.[5]

Failure to provide pain relief during a preimplantation trial may occur for several reasons: test injections made in the wrong place; psychological reasons such as depression; advanced tolerance to opioids; incorrect dose of spinal drugs; or a principal component of the patient's symptoms being not susceptible to spinal application of opioid (e.g. some central pain syndromes).[4] If a question remains about the ability of spinal drugs to provide symptom relief after two trial doses, a placebo injection may help clarify the situation.

It is widely accepted that this response to acute drug administration is highly predictive of the long-term outcome of chronic drug administration. Failure to see adequate, long-lasting analgesia under these conditions is cause to reconsider placement of an implantable narcotic-delivery system.

Unless the efficacy of spinal opioids is clearly demonstrated during the preimplantation trial, the patient could be subjected to the implantation of a delivery system that will fail to achieve the desired pain relief. With the exception of electrical stimulation and spinal drugs, few invasive pain therapies allow the patient and physician to test the therapy before an irreversible result has occurred. Local anaesthetic blocks are useful in educating the patient before neurodestructive procedures but cannot always predict the adequacy, extent, or complications of an irreversible destructive procedure.

Infection and local conditions

Infection, inflammation, or dermatitis at the proposed cutaneous site of implantation—and the presence of generalised sepsis—represent absolute contraindications to device implantation.

Anticoagulation and haematological abnormalities

The fully anticoagulated patient represents a special problem when considering placement of an implantable drug-delivery system. Pre-implantation trials of spinal drugs for the relief of pelvic and lower body pain have been performed safely in the presence of anticoagulation by administering the opioid caudally with a 25 gauge, 1·5 inch needle.[6] Unfortunately, spinal opioids administered in the lumbar or caudal region may not relieve upper body pain without a substantial increase in the dose. Carefully weigh the risk-to-benefit ratio of stopping anticoagulants in order to proceed with preimplantation trials of cervical or thoracic spinal drugs.

Coagulopathy caused by disease is also common, particularly in cancer patients. Platelet count and function, and tests for procoagulant factor activity should be assessed in all cancer patients and others whose history or physical examination suggests the possibility of coagulopathy. Efforts should be made to reverse the coagulopathy if possible. If this is not possible, assess the risk-to-benefit ratio of proceeding with preimplantation trials.

Physiological abnormalities

Physiological abnormalities, such as electrolyte imbalance and drug-induced organic brain syndrome, may impair the patient's ability to assess the adequacy of symptom relief.[4] Many abnormalities are reversible and an effort should be made to correct them before a trial of spinal drugs is undertaken. It should be remembered that the confusion secondary to these physiological abnormalities may be incorrectly interpreted as uncontrolled pain by the patient and pain management specialist alike.

Behavioural abnormalities

Behavioural abnormalities that are often difficult to identify may affect the patient's ability to assess the adequacy of symptom relief. These abnormalities may coexist with physiological factors but care must be taken not to attribute inadequate symptom relief solely to behavioural factors until all potential physiological causes have been explored.[7]

Support system

An implantable drug-delivery system requires a level of commitment from patients, and their support systems. Someone must be available day and night to care for and inject the implantable drug-delivery system should the patient be unable to do so. Thus one or more persons must be designated as the patient's support system for implantable drug-delivery systems, and these individuals must be acceptable to the patient. It should be remembered that cancer patients who are able to inject their own implantable drug-delivery systems initially may be unable to do so later in the course of disease. Inability or unwillingness by the designated support system to care for the implantable drug-delivery system has signifcant implications when selecting the appropriate system.

Life expectancy

Although prediction of a cancer patient's life expectancy can be difficult, an estimate in terms of days, weeks, or months is essential to select the most appropriate implantable drug-delivery system.[1] Often the patient's general condition wil improve when adequate symptom control is provided, and this must be taken into account when estimating life expectancy.

Types of implantable drug-delivery systems

Type I percutaneous catheters

The Type I percutaneous catheters have gained wide acceptance for the short term administration of spinal opioids and/or local anaesthetics for the palliation of acute pain, including obstetric and postoperative pain. The Type I system also has three applications in cancer pain management. The first is in the acute setting, where delivery of opioids into the epidural or subarachnoid space can provide temporary palliation of pain post-operatively or until other concurrent treatments, such as radiotherapy, become effective. The second is in imminently dying patients too ill for more invasive procedures.[148] The third is in the use of a percutaneous catheter to administer test doses of spinal opioids before placing a more permanent implantable drug-delivery system. In many centres the use of a Type I percutaneous catheter to deliver epidural, and especially sub-arachnoid opioids, is limited. Improved catheter fixation, reduced risk of infection, and the relative ease of tunnelling[139] has led many pain specialists to tunnel the spinal catheter to the flank, abdomen or chest wall, even for the short term administration of opioids. Despite several reports that the Type I system can be used for prolonged periods in immunocompromised patients without an increased risk of infection,[10] the validity of this observation has not been established. In view of the potentially devastating and life-threatening consequences of catheter-induced spinal infection, as well as the highly favourable risk-to-benefit ratio of the Type II tunnelled catheter, the use of the Type I system should be limited solely to the acute setting.

Type II subcutaneous tunnelled catheters

The subcutaneous tunnelled catheters are selected for patients with life expectancies of weeks to months. The low cost, ease of implementation, and ease of catheter care and injection make the Type II system the preferred delivery system at many centres. The Type II system can be implanted or removed in the outpatient setting, and has a decreased incidence of infection when compared with the Type I system.

Type III totally implantable reservoir

The totally implantable reservoir is often chosen for patients with life expectancies of months to years who have had excellent relief of symptoms with trial doses of spinal drugs.[110] The Type III system has potentially less risk of infection than Type I and II systems, and a decreased risk of catheter failure. Injection of the Type III system is more difficult than with Type I and II systems; this can be significant when training lay people to inject and care for this system.[11] Furthermore, removal or replacement requires a surgical incision.

Type IV totally implantable mechanically activated pump

Poletti and colleagues created one of the earliest totally implantable systems for patient-activated drug delivery. This system consisted of an implantable sterile blood bag with a hydrocephalus shunt valve in series with the bag and spinal catheter. The valve could be activated by the patient to allow self-administration of an opioid from the implanted bag. This concept has now been extended by Cordis, through introduction of a totally implantable reservoir that is accessed percutaneously through a septum on the surface of the device. The device also has a mechanical valve system activated by a set of buttons on the pump surface. The patient delivers spinal drugs by depressing the buttons in the proper sequence.[1] The Type IV system has potentially less risk of infection than the Types I, II and III systems. Subarachnoid delivery is more feasible with the Type IV system than with Type I and II systems. The greatest advantage of this system is that the patient can titrate the dose of the drug based on symptoms, and can pretreat symptoms prior to periods of increased activity

Type V totally implantable infusion pump

The totally implantable infusion pump is also used in patients with life expectancies of months to years who obtained relief of symptoms after trial doses of spinal drugs.[1 12] Type V delivery systems may also be indicated in cancer patients with shorter life expectancies, who experience intermittent confusion secondary to metabolic abnormalities or systematically administered drugs. Clinical experience suggests that such patients may obtain analgesia with fewer side-effects with low dose continuous spinal opioid infusion than repeated bolus injections into a spinal catheter. Alternatively, an implanted port with an external infusion pump may suffice in this situation, although this may be more inconvenient and require more support.

Since Type V systems require infrequent refills, and run continuously, they are ideal for patients with limited medical or non-medical family support services. The Type V system is usually selected with an auxiliary bolus injection port to take advantage of potential drug options, such as local anaesthetic injections.

Advantages of the Type V system include the minimal risk of infection after the perioperative period, and the infrequent need to inject the pump relative to other implantable drug-delivery systems where the pump reservoir needs to be refilled approximately every 7–20 days. The overall high cost of the Type V system is a disadvantage and may occasionally result in selecting a less effective or more inconvenient analgesic technique.

Type VI totally implantable programmable infusion pump

The Type VI totally implantable programmable infusion pump is implanted with the same ease as the Type V system.[13] This system allows a broad spectrum of delivery rates and modes, including occasional bolus injections. Its principal application to date has been intrathecal infusion, especially in the therapy of spasticity in multiple sclerosis and spinal cord-injured patients.[13 14] There is yet no proved advantage of programmable systems over the simpler continuous infusion systems. However, there are several theoretical advantages for cancer pain patients, including the reduction of side-effects that may occur with the bolus injections provided by Types I, II, III and IV implantable drug-delivery systems, coupled with the added ability to pretreat symptoms associated with periods of increased activity.

Subcutaneous placement of epidural catheters for long term administration

In patients who require long term administration of intaspinal narcotics, the subcutaneously implanted delivery systems offer the safest option. Silastic catheters are preferable to catheters made of other materials because they cause less tissue reaction when implanted on a long term basis. Tissue reaction has been implicated in the development of tolerance to intraspinal narcotics. A variety of silastic catheters small enough to allow placement through a 17 gauge Tuohy needle are now commercially available. Many of these catheters are sold with a malleable tunnelling device. The malleability of the tunnelling device also allows for tunnelling the catheter around the flank without repeated in and out manoeuvres that may increase the risk of infection or catheter damage.

The technique is suitable for the patient who is suffering from severe multisystem disease and may not be a candidate for more invasive procedures. The anaesthetist may perform this technique on an outpatient basis, which avoids the inconvenience, risk, and expense of hospitalisation. Subcutaneous placement of silastic catheters offers a simple, safe, and cost-effective approach to the long term delivery of intraspinal narcotics.

Neural stimulation: spinal cord and peripheral nerve stimulation

Neural stimulation has been a significant part of medical history. Advances in today's technology and physiological research have helped define avenues where this tool, when properly used, can afford society outstanding clinical and economic benefits.

The first multiprogrammable electronics were introduced in 1980, and totally implantable neural stimulator systems were introduced in 1981.

Eight-channel multiprogammable electronics and the first eight-electrode catheter were developed in 1986. Following this, 1988 signalled the introduction of the non-invasive programmable implantable pulse generator that also had radiofrequency capabilities. In the 1990s, successful adaptation of multilead electrode arrays, implantable programmmable pulse generators, implantable radiofrequency receivers, and more sophisticated objective patient screening methods, has led to very high success rates.

Physiology

The sensitivity of neural tissue to frequency and amplitude variations significantly alters the physiological response in the living organism. High frequency, low amplitude stimulation silences most dorsal horn cells, including presumably noxious ones, which are active only during strong pinching or clamping. The inhibition is dramatic. Conversely, low frequency, high amplitude stimulation is much less effective. This may explain part of the efficacy of spinal cord stimulation or peripheral nerve stimulation for peripheral vascular disease and reflex sympathetic dystrophy, since sympathetic fibres are normally recruited more with this type of stimulation. Inhibition of the sympathetic system is more likely by high frequency, low amplitude stimulation.

Stimulation recruits Aβ-fibres; paraesthesia is frequently dependent. If a patient is stimulated at higher freqeuncies, Aδ-fibres are recruited and the frequency dependency is diminished. Excess Aδ-fibre stimulation causes the patient to report unpleasant paraesthesia, which might feel prickling or even epicritic (sharp, well localised). However, if such a paraesthesia was better able to suppress C-fibre activity, then pain would be less protopathic (agonal, diffuse).

Stimulating large diameter afferents with non-noxious stimuli could close down or inhibit messages from the ascending small diameter nociceptive fibres and interneurons. Subsequent theories include inhibitory pathways being stimulated by spinal descending tracts. Spinal cord stimulation physiologically may be affected by a number of mechanisms. The basics include electrical contact with a cathode (negative electrode), which causes excitation of nervous tissue. The inside of living neural cells is negatively charged. Thus the exposure of an external negative charge causes depolarisation to a positive potential on the inside of the cell, which therefore causes an action potential and thus a non-noxious message.

Chronic pain sufferers have demonstrated lower levels of endorphin and serotonin in the CSF when compared to subjects who did not complain of chronic pain. Both chemicals show demonstrative increases that are subject to neural stimulation, although the analgesic effects of spinal cord stimulation have not been reversible by naloxone.[15]

Indications

The general indications for spinal cord stimulation are for suppression of chronic, intractable pain of the trunk or limbs.[16] Examples of specific diseases where spinal cord stimulation may be indicated include: arachnoiditis[17]; spastic torticollis; intercostal neuralgia; peripheral neuropathy[18]; reflex sympathetic dystrophy[19]; phantom limb pain[20]; radicular pain associated with intraspinal fibrosis; peripheral pain associated with ischaemic vascular disease[21]; and peripheral pain associated with postherpetic neuralgia.

Certain conditions that are specifically amenable to peripheral nerve stimulation include reflex sympathetic dystrophy, causalgia, direct nerve injury, and plexus avulsion. The pathologies that respond best to peripheral stimulation are deafferentation or neuropathic conditions.

Conditions for implantation

Guidelines have been established by the Health Care and Finance Administration (HCFA) on implantation of spinal cord and peripheral nerve stimulators. Spinal cord stimulators should be used only:

1 As a late resort for patients with chronic, intractable pain
2 When other treatment modalities (pharmacological, surgical, physical, or psychological therapies) have been tried and do not prove satisfactory, have been judged to be unsuitable, or contraindicated for the patient
3 When patients have undergone careful screening and diagnosis by a multidisciplinary team before implantation
4 When all the facilities, equipment, and professional support personnel required for the proper diagnosis, treatment, training, and follow-up of the patient are available
5 When demonstration of pain relief with a *temporarily implanted* electrode precedes permanent implantation
6 With demonstrated pathology (an objective basis for the pain)
7 With documentation of no drug addiction.

The screening criteria for peripheral nerve stimulation, including the previous guidelines, should also include pain confined or related to a specific nerve branch, and pain that can be ablated by a peripheral nerve block. This will be discussed in more detail later.

Contraindications

There are a few relative contraindications to spinal cord stimulation as a therapeutic option:

1 Patient fails the screening
2 Patient is adverse to electrical stimulation
3 Patient is adverse to an implant as a modality of treating their pain

4 An active and uncontrolled coagulopathy at the time of the planned procedure

5 Diffuse distribution of pain is localised or disseminated at the time of the planned implantation

6 Physician's lack of experience or training in implanting stimulator devices

7 Patient has a demand cardiac pacemaker

8 Patient needs MRI in the immediate foreseeable future

9 Untreated and unresolved serious drug habituation

10 Absence of an objectively documented cause for pain.

Failed treatment

It is extremely important to document, within the confines of the history and physical examination, what medications and therapeutic interventions have not been successful for the patient. Specifically indicate the medical, neurosurgical, orthopaedic, vascular, behavioural medicine, or other consultants who have been involved. Determine that there are contra-indications to spinal cord implantation and that no better alternatives exist.

Implantation procedures

Precautions

The screening stimulator lead array is implanted in a sterile operating room. Determine that adequate stimulation has been achieved on the operating room table. The stimulator paraesthesia must cover the area of pain if at all possible. The entire system is not implanted in a single setting. The possible exception to this is in cases of objective documentation of clinical improvement in peripheral vascular disease. Operating room screening and immediate full system implantation is discouraged for the following reasons:

1 The patient is usually under the influence of a preoperative or intraoperative sedative administered to ease their discomfort during the placement of the intraspinal lead.

2 The patient is not hearing during the time of lead implantation and is not participating. Thus using a stimulator system is an unrealistic test of pain relief.

3 The transient changes in body chemistry and position may remove the pain generator. Therefore the physician may not have the opportunity to see the pain in its most exaggerated form during the brief tenure in the operating room.

Ambulation after temporary placement of the lead in the prone or lateral position may cause migration of a percutaneously placed lead, thus altering the area of stimulation. Be certain that the system to be implanted can withstand changing positions from recumbent to ambulatory, and make sure that the paraesthesia coverage does not vary significantly with ambulation.

It is recommended that the patient receives intravenous prophylaxis antibiotic approximately 30 minutes before the percutaneous implantation of the lead array. It is recommended that, without exception, all leads be placed with fluoroscopic guidance. A mild sedative should be available to patients to help lessen the trauma of the experience of having a spinal cord stimulating electrode placed into the spinal canal, and to diminish the probability of sudden dangerous movement.

Procedure

The patient should be maintained on antibiotics as long as the percutaneous lead is present, and for a brief period subsequent to total system implantation. The decision whether to place an implantable programmable neurological stimulator power source or a radiofrequency receiver with external transmitter and antennae is based on a number of variables. The first and foremost is whether the physics of the implanted system are exceeded during the screening period. Other factors to consider include the use of the external power source depending on the patient being able to place their antennae somewhere, if the system is guided by an audible signal. This may cause problems with patients who have impaired hearing. The problem can be overcome by teaching patients to find their radiofrequency receiver by a shrinking concentric circle motion until they reach maximal stimulation from the antennae.

Once the patient is capable of properly operating the system, he or she is discharged, usually within 12–24 hours of the final implant.

Peripheral nerve stimulation

Peripheral nerve stimulation has been used since 1965. Peripheral nerve stimulation was initially performed with cuffs containing stimulation electrodes. Technical and clinical complications were significant. Electrode migration and equipment malfunction created the need for more stable equipment design to be developed. Scar formation caused by direct contact between the nerve and the cuff led to nerve constriction. Flat electrode arrays with a thin panel of fascia between the nerve and the stimulator proved to be much more stable and clinically effective.[22]

Peripheral nerve stimulation has been used successfully to treat pain of neurogenic origin in upper extremities, lower extemities, and intercostal nerves. As equipment design improved so did the clinical selection and screening procedure.

Selection criteria for peripheral nerve stimulation

Patients with single nerve pathology are the best peripheral nerve stimulator candidates. Patients with multiple nerve lesions have been successfully screened and implanted. Clinical syndromes that have responded favourably to peripheral nerve stimulation include:

- Reflex sympathetic dystrophy
- Causalgia
- Plexus avulsion
- Operative trauma
- Entrapment neuropathies
- Injection injuries.

Clinical selection criteria include:

- Chronic intractable pain, recalcitant to other therapies
- Temporary relief from local anaesthetic injection
- No psychological contraindications
- Objective evidence of pathology (e.g. electromyography, somatosensory evoked potential, or selective tissue conductance studies)
- No drug habituation
- Relief from temporary screen.

Complications

Patient-related complications might include infection, bleeding, adverse drug reaction, injury to the spinal cord, nerve injury, CSF leak, poor pain relief, fibrosis at the tip of the stimulator, and/or motor stimulation. Mechanical problems that may occur include lead fracture, lead shearing and shortage, intraoperative or postoperative lead movement, extension cable fracture, battery malfunction or depletion, or transmitter malfunction or depletion.

Efficacy

Spinal cord stimulation has been reported in 53–70% of patients over 2·2–5 years. Reports to measure the effectiveness of spinal cord stimulation include: good to excellent pain relief, decreased consumption of narcotics and other analgesics, improved tissue oxygenation, decreased incidence of amputation in peripheral vascular disease, increased activities of daily living, and return to work.

Radiofrequency

Electrical current has been used to produce neural lesions in patients for 100 years. Modern radiofrequency thermocoagulation has been used to ablate pain pathways in the trigeminal ganglion, spinal cord, dorsal root entry zone, DRG, sympathetic chain, and peripheral nerves. Unfortunately, the long term effects of ablative techniques on clinical pain syndromes are incompletely known.

The radiofrequency lesion is formed when neural temperature exceeds 45°C. These temperatures are a result of frictional heat that is generated by molecular movement in a field of alternating current at radiowave frequency. Frequencies above 250 kHz produce an electromagnetic field around an active electrode. An active electrode is placed in the desired anatomical location, and an indifferent electrode is placed to minimise current passage across the myocardium. The current disperses via the second electrode, which is usually a high area contact plate. Wattage is gradually increased, and heat develops in the tissue, which conducts to the active probe. Heat is generated as current flows through a probe with a built-in thermocouple. Thus the thermocouple needle combination allows lesioning, monitoring and injecting without movement of the appropriately positioned device. The temperature of the probe itself assumes equilibrium with the temperature of the tissue surrounding it. The heat is not emitted from the probe itself but from the current movement which generates the heat as it passes through the tissues. The temperture is monitored, and wattage is adjusted to a target temperature, which is a primary determinant of lesion size. For low power procedures such as facet denervation, 10–20 watts are used. Other factors such as active electrode diameter and length contribute to wattage requirements. Tissue blood flow is important because significant heat convection can occur, with significant blood flow in the area of the lesion. Homogeneous tissue is necessary for a lesion shape that is symmetrical.[23]

Efficacy

Radiofrequency lesioning is a neurodestructive procedure. Therefore it has to be considered an end-of-the-line procedure where conservative therapeutic modalities have failed. The physician performing radio-frequency procedures must have appropriate training and experience before beginning such neurodestructive procedures. All of these procedures should be done under fluoroscopic guidance after appropriate test stimulation and verification of the tissues about to be destroyed has been accomplished. Different temperatures have various levels of neurodestructive capabilities. Numbness or motor paralysis occurs very rarely as a consequence of the lesioning. The tissues can be injured anywhere along the passing of the needle probe if there is a break in the insulation. Therefore supermaximal motor stimulation is always part of the procedure before lesioning is performed, in the event that the insulated portion of the needle passes near a motor nerve such as in lumbar sympathetic lesioning. If there is a break in insulation, not only the lumbar sympathetic ganglion but also the lumbar nerve root may be neurodestructed, which is definitely not the desired outcome. Kline[34] described the essential information for trainees and others interested in radiofrequency techniques.

Radiofrequency lesioning can have definite advantages over alternative neurodestructive procedures, primarily because the lesion is controlled. The complications associated with neurolytic solutions, resulting from intravascular injection and spread along tissue planes, can be avoided. The proximal and distal spread of the lesion beyond the uninsulated tip of the probe is only 1 mm, and the cross-sectional diameter of the lesion is 5–6 mm. The advantages include:[24]

1 Well-controlled lesion size
2 Temperature is monitored in the core of the lesion by the built-in thermocouple
3 Electrode placement can be verified by fluoroscopic guidance using electrical stimulation and impedance monitoring
4 Procedure can be performed without general anaesthetics
5 Procedure can be performed on an outpatient basis, and effectiveness can be recognised in approximately 4 weeks
6 There is low morbidity and mortality associated with the lesioning itself; however, potential complications include major neurological injury, and extreme care must be taken when injecting local anaesthetic and steroids, as well as during probe placement, location verification, and lesion formation
7 Procedure can be repeated.

Monitor patients because radiofrequency equipment can interact with pacemakers and spinal cord stimulators. The equipment used in the procedure must be safe, precise, and yield reproducible results. The equipment[24] must be able to:

1 Measure impedance
2 Stimulate a wide range of frequencies
3 Accurately time the duration of the lesion for precise temperature measurement in the core of the lesion tissue
4 Accurately measure and indicate amperage and voltage
5 Gradually increase temperature with time.

Patient selection should be selected based on the following criteria:[24]

1 Other non-invasive conservative measures have failed.
2 Substance abuse has been identified and dealt with, such as opioids, sedatives, and alcohol; the patient has entered a programme to resolve the issues in addition to symptom control.
3 Appropriate psychological assessment and therapy has been performed for depression, anxiety, anger, and secondary gain; the patient has been entered into an appropriate behavioural management programme.

4 The patient accepts his/her lifestyle changes, addresses psychological issues, and interacts with physicians, therapists and psychologists in an appropriate manner.

5 Fully informed consent, including recognition of realistic expectations and procedural risks, must be obtained.

Procedural considerations must be preceded by full awareness of the anatomy, pain pathways, anticipated outcomes, and the need to have a multidisciplinary team around the individual carrying out such procedures.

The most commonly used procedures include neurodestructive procedures around facet joints in the neck, thoracic, lumbar, and lumbar cervical areas. Anterior compartment pain from lumbar disease can be solved by lesioning the anterior communicating branch.[25] Radiofrequency lumbar ganglionotomy, partial rhizotomy, sacral ganglionotomy, thoracic ganglionotomy, cervical ganglionotomy, cervical facets, discs, nerve roots, myofascial tissues, sphenopalatine ganglion, and radiofrequency lesioning of the stellate ganglion via the interior approach, have been quite useful at C6, C7, and TL areas.

Radiofrequency lesioning of the trigeminal ganglion, as described by Sweet, has been an important technique in neurosurgical circles.[26] Percutaneous cordotomy is probably the most studied and indicated procedure, and especially affects the torso on the contralateral side of the lesioning. The hazards of the procedure include worse pain when the patient outlives the duration of the lesioning, and the possibility of Ordine's curse if bilateral lesioning is carried out. The incidence of radiofrequency cordotomies, even in patients with cancer pain, seems to have decreased since the introduction of spinal opioids, other neuroaugmentation procedures such as spinal cord stimulation, and in patients who respond favourably to more modern forms of cancer therapies. It is especially tragic when complications of therapy such as permanent numbness or, in rare instances, development of neuropathic pain persist when the cancer is no longer a problem. As a general rule, deafferentation pains do not respond to radiofrequency lesioning.

Cryolysis

Cryoanalgesia is a term for creating a nerve injury by freezing. Cryoanalgesia developments include: carbon dioxide and fashioning into dry ice pencils for topical application; cooling metal rods (cryoprobes) in baths of dry ice and acetone or ether, and pressing the rods against the tissue to be frozen.

It was not until liquid air and liquid nitrogen became available, however that another generation of more powerful cryoprobes was developed. In 1961 Cooper and colleagues developed the first cryoprobe.[27] The probe employed the principle of phase change using liquid nitrogen to produce a temperature of $-196°C$. Later, Amoils developed a smaller, more easily controlled probe for ophthalmic surgery, and introduced the enclosed gas expansion cryoprobe.[28] This probe, which used the Joule-Thompson principle, was driven by liquid carbon dioxide, and was capable of reaching temperatures of $-50°C$. Since that time, numerous probes have been developed using this principle and nitrous oxide as the primary refrigerant, which is capable of achieving minimal temperatures of approximately $-70°C$. Currently, these probes are available in many sizes and shapes and have incorporated thermocouples and nerve stimulators. Many probes can be inserted through the skin for localisation and freezing of nerves percutaneously.[29]

Nelson and colleagues,[30] Brain,[31] and Lloyd and colleagues[29] applied cryoprobes to various nerves, including intercostal, pharyngeal, trigeminal, sacral and others in the treatment of various chronic neuralgias and pain. Lloyd and his colleagues are credited with naming the technique cryoanalgesia, and have demonstrated that prolonged analgesia can be obtained after a single freeze of a peripheral nerve. They particularly stressed the safety of the procedure and reported that nerve function always returned and neuroma formation did not occur.[29]

Histological basis of cryoneurolysis

The mechanism of cold-induced nerve injury is still unknown. Many explanations have been suggested, including: hypertonicity of intracellular and extracellular fluids, physical destruction by large cellular ice crystals, minimal cell volume, damage to proteins, membrane rupture caused by rapid water loss, ischaemic necrosis, and the production of autoantibodies. Many of the studies have been conducted *in vitro*, and subsequent interpretation is difficult. However, freezing represents nothing more than the removal of pure water from a solution and isolating it as ice crystals into an inert foreign body. All subsequent biochemical, anatomical and physiological consequences of freezing are directly or indirectly the consequence of this single event. Many have closely studied the mechanism of freeze injury, and they all agreed that the major factors in freeze injury were the development of intracellular and extracellular ice crystals.[32] The formation of ice either causes gross shifts in tissue osmolarity and cell wall permeability or produces physical disruption of the myelin sheath and Schwann's cell.[32] It has been pointed out that freezing an injury also caused extensive vascular damage and permitted plasma and extracellular extravasation, which increased endoneural fluid pressure. Subsequently, they found that the nerve fibre underwent wallerian degeneration, a process associated with elevated endoneural fluid pressure. Nevertheless, once the ice crystal formation produced destruction of the nerve, no additional benefit was achieved by decreasing the temperatue of the cell. However, it was found that the size of the lesion created and the length of nerve involvement were temperature dependent to a point.[32]

Sunderland described categories or "degrees" of peripheral nerve injury based on histology and prognosis.[33] The degree of injury sought by a peripheral cryolesion is that of a second-degree injury, which occurs when a short length of peripheral nerve is frozen to −20°C or lower. In this injury, there is a "loss of axonal continuity without breaching of the endoneurium". The axons of nerve are damaged at the site of injury. The fibrous architecture (endoneurium, perineurium, epineurium) of the nerve, however, is preserved. The axon and the myelin sheaths degenerate from the point of freezing distally to the nerve's termination (wallerian degeneration). Regeneration begins immediately from the proximal stump. The growing tips of individual axons (growth cones) advance distally within the lumen of their still intact endoneural tubes at a rate of approximately 1·0–1·5 mm per day. After a period of time, and a distance directly proportional from the point of injury to the distal end of the nerve, axon sprouts reach their end organs. Nerve histology after regrowth is restored to normal. However, maximum nerve conduction velocity remains reduced on average 35 days, even after new myelin sheaths have fully matured.[34] However, normal sensory and motor functions do return, provided that (in the case of limbs) regrowth occurs before irreversible endoneural fibrosis, muscle wasting, or contractures can occur.

Third-, fourth- and fifth-degree injuries occur with more permanent forms of neurolytic lesions, such as the use of radiofrequency thermocoagulation, alcohol, phenol, and surgical resection. These types of nerve injuries are prone to neuritis and the formation of neuromas. Because of the disruption of the endoneural and perineural fibre sheaths, respectively, there is a more erratic and disorganised reformation of the nerve between the nerve stump and its end organ. Useful regeneration does not occur with fifth-degree injuries; the nerve is completely transected, and the two ends are separated. Neuromas, however, can still form.

In contrast, a cryolesion is reversible and has not been associated with neuromas. In several studies on animals, there is no evidence of neuroma formation at necropsy, and the degree of fibrosis and scarring at the site of injury is minimal. The extent of cell destruction by a cryolesion will depend on several factors, but the rate of freezing and thawing and the temperature attained by the tissue in proximity to the cryoprobe are the most important.[32] Evans and coworkers showed that when a rat sciatic nerve was directly exposed to cryoneurolysis, the time for regeneration of the nerve was independent of the duration of freezing and the application of a repeat freeze cycle.[32] However, the temperature attained by the nerve is important. Evans concluded that where the temperature remained greater than −20°C, the results are unpredictable. Below this temperature, the interruption was prolonged and uninfluenced by greater reductions in temperature.[32]

When using a percutaneous cryoprobe, the rate of cooling the tissue depends on the geometry of the cryoprobe and its capacity for heat extraction. The "iceball" (probe tip to ice interface with tissue) shows a sharp temperature gradient across its radius of approximately 10°C/ml. The tissues closest to the probe attain the maximum sub-zero temperature, whereas the remaining tissues show a rapid rise toward 0°C. The central zone undergoes rapid cooling while the peripheral zone is influenced by the heat generated as the surrounding tissue slowly cools. Extending the duration of freezing will produce some increase in the size of the iceball and the central zone until a plateau is reached, whereby heat extraction by the probe balances the heat production by the surrounding tissue. Here again, Gill and coworkers showed that repetitive freezing could increase the amount of tissue frozen and the rate of freezing tissue surrounding the probe. Despite debate in the literature, there is uniform agreement that below − 20°C causes cellular freezing, and cells do not recover.

Structure of the cryoprobe

Modern versions of the cryoprobe also utilise a temperature thermocouple embedded in the tip to measure the probe temperature. A nerve stimulator is also incorporated to help freeze pinpoint nerves and to avoid those nerves not intended to be lysed. The typical freeze-zone diameter for a gas expansion cryoprobe set at − 60°C is two to three times the probe's diameter, as compared with 3·5–5·0 times the diameter of a liquid nitrogen probe at − 180°C. The standard freeze zone that could be created at equilibrium was approximately 10 mm with the 14 gauge gas expansion cryoprobe, and approximately 6 mm with the 16 gauge cryoprobe, as measured by the author *in vitro*.

The second type of cryoprobe uses a change of phase to produce refrigeration. The original model was designed in 1951 by Irving Cooper and Arnold Lee, and that basic design continued to be followed today. Their design consisted of a long insulated metal tube through which a stream of liquid nitrogen could enter and evaporate.

Temperatures of − 196°C can be attained with a liquid nitrogen cryoprobe. Freezing capacity is proportional to the rate at which liquid nitrogen is delivered to the surface area of the probe tip, and the rate at which latent heat evaporates the liquid nitrogen.

Recently, a helium gas cryoprobe has been described. The construction is similar to the liquid nitrogen probe, but it uses helium gas that has been precooled to − 80°C by liquid nitrogen. This cold gas is delivered at a high velocity to impinge on the spherically shaped probe tip. The gas is then redirected back through the annulus surrounding the supply tube.[35] Bald reported that an 8 mm probe tip created an iceball of 28 mm at 10 minutes of freezing with a gas flow of 42 litres/min and a tip temperature of − 138°C. The clinical utility for this probe remains to be seen.

Specific lesions with percutaneous cryoprobe

Percutaneous cryoprobe application has been used for many types of neural lesioning. In fact, any nerve that can be isolated by percutaneous or direct vision cryoprobe can undergo cryoneurolysis. The following is a review of some of the more popular uses for the cryoprobe. However, despite the lack of neuroma formation and low incidence of neuritis with a cryolesion, it is not a benign procedure, and cryoneurolysis of motor nerves should be avoided.

Facial pain

Treatment of postherpetic and non-herpetic trigeminal neuralgia by cryoneurolysis has been described throughout the literature. Barnard *et al* also described the use of cryoneurolysis for post-traumatic neuralgia, malignant disease causing facial pain, and neuralgia of unknown aetiology. They used the cryoprobe to lyse supraorbital, supratrochlear, infraorbital, mental, and lingual nerves in 21 patients. In these patients, they compared freezing followed by sectioning to freezing alone. They found that the median time of pain relief was 116 days for cryoneurolysis alone and only 38 days for freezing and subsequent sectioning. However, sensory loss lasted 49 days for cryoneurolyis and 131 days for freezing and sectioning. They concluded that cryoanalgesia was a useful therapeutic tool for the management of intractable facial pain because it provided a reliable, prolonged, and reversible nerve block that could be achieved by a simple technique that did not appear to aggravate symptoms.[36] Goss described using cryoneurotomy for intractable temporomandibular joint pain. In his review of six consecutive patients with intractable neurogenic pain of the auricular nerves, cryoneurolysis was performed percutaneously, and all six patients had excellent pain relief for 1 year after the procedure. Four of the six had recurrent pain. He also found that repeat cryoneurolysis had decreasing effectiveness.[37] Cryoprobes have also been described for use in oral surgry and pituitary cryoablation.[38]

Thoracic pain

Chronic and acute thoracic pain have been treated with cryoneurolysis, intraoperatively at the end of thoracotomy for acute pain and percutaneously for chronic thoracic pain.

Spinal pain

The use of the percutaneous cryoprobe for facet rhizotomy has also been described in the literature for the treatment of low back pain and the lumbar disc syndrome. This procedure is used to block the articular nerve of Luschka at the junction of the pedicle with the transverse process. At this site, the nerve has not yet branched into its ascending, lateral and medial branches; therefore a single lesion can produce analgesia. However, in this technique, the nerve may be lysed at the level in question, at one level above, and one level below the facet of pathology. This is due to the branching nature of the nerves innervating the facets. Schuster used this technique for treating facet pain in 52 patients and found that 47 of these patients had significant relief from back pain. Of these 47, only one had to be returned for recurrent pain after 9 months without pain.[39]

Pelvic pain

Sacral foramenal cryolesions have also been used to treat cancer, coccydynia, and sciatic pain. A bilateral S4 block is useful for treating coccydynia and perineal pain from cancer of the rectum; reportedly, this avoids bladder denervation. Also, S1 and S2 cryolesions can treat pain in sciatic distribution. However, multiple bilateral sacral block is best avoided in view of the possibility of bladder dysfunction as a complication.

Cryoneurolysis of the iliohypogastric and ilioinguinal nerves has also been described. In a study by Khiroya et al, cryoneurolysis of the ilioinguinal nerve was performed for postoperative pain relief after herniorrhaphy.[40] These authors compared patients who had their ilioinguinal nerves frozen during surgery with those who did not, and they concluded that cryoanalgesia of the ilioinguinal nerve alone did not produce significant early postherniorrhaphy pain relief.

Peripheral nerve pain

Blocking peripheral nerves by cryotherapy has been used for neuroma, causalgia, flexion contractures, and nerve entrapment syndromes. The nerves to be frozen must not have a significant motor component unless motor destruction is the goal; for example, in the later stages of multiple sclerosis. The reversibility of the nerve block, however, allows for return of motor function after normal regeneration. Wang reported that, in patients treated for chronically painful peripheral nerve lesions, 50% of the patients treated in one study had pain relief for 1–12 months.[41] He also reported that the pain eventually returned. However, during the period of remission, patients returned to normal activities. Wang concurred with the concept that it is especially important when freezing peripheral nerves to have precise localisation of the nerves in order to obtain adequate neurolysis.

Complications of cryotherapy

Many of the complications reported in the literature pertain to the use of cutaneous cryosurgery. With this technique the nerves will be affected and

217

may cause persistent pain. To prevent this as much as possible, cryosurgical equipment must be tested thoroughly before using to ensure that there are no leaks. A significant leakage of refrigerant can cause freezing along the shaft of the cryoprobe and subsequent freezing of structures other than those intended.

The most common problem is frostbite of the skin at the entry site, which can usually be prevented by an introducer sheath. Unattended motor damage can occur, but the patient very often recovers. A frustrating aspect of cryoneurolysis is that therapeutic effectiveness cannot be predicted; pain relief can last from 3 to 1000 days.

References

1 Waldman SD, Coombs DW. Selection of implantable narcotic delivery systems. *Anesth Analg* 1989;**68**:377–84.
2 Waldman SD, Cronen MC. Thoracic epidural morphine in the palliation of chest wall pain secondary to relapsing polychondritis. *J Pain Symptom Management* 1989;**4**:60–3.
3 Waldman SD. A simplified approach to the subcutaneous placement of epidural catheters for long-term administration of morphine sulfate. *J Pain Symptom Management* 1987;**3**:163–6.
4 Waldman SD, Feldstein GS, Allen ML. Selection of patients for implantable spinal narcotic delivery systems. *Anesth Analg* 1986;**65**:883–5.
5 Coombs DW, Saunders RL, Schweberger CL. Epidural narcotic infusion reservoir: implantation technique and efficacy. *Anesthesiology* 1982;**56**:469–73.
6 Waldman SD, Feldstein GS, Waldman HJ, *et al.* Caudal administration of morphine sulfate in anticoagulated and thrombocytopenic patients. *Anesth Analg* 1987;**66**:267–8.
7 Zenz M. Epidural opiates for the treatment of cancer pain. In: Zimmerman M, Drugs P, Wagner G, eds, *Recent results in cancer research.* Heidelberg: Springer-Verlag, 1989:107–15.
8 Crawford ME, Anderson HB, Augustenborg G, *et al.* Pain treatment on outpatient basis utilizing extradural opiates: a Danish multicenter study comprising 105 patients. *Pain* 1983;**16**:41–6.
9 Peder C, Crawford M. Fixation of epidural catheters by means of subcutaneous tissue tunneling. *Ugeskr Laeger* 1982;**144**:2631–3.
10 Downing JE, Busch EH, Stedman PM. Epidural morphine delivered by a percutaneous epidural catheter for outpatient treatment of cancer pain. *Anesth Analg* 1988;**67**:1159–61.
11 Cousin M, Gourley G, Cherry D. A technique for the insertion of an implantable portal system for the long-term epidural administration of opioids in the treatment of cancer pain. *Anesth Intensive Care* 1985;**13**:145–52.
12 Gestin Y. A totally implantable multi-dose pump allowing cancer patients intrathecal access for the self-administration of morphine at home: a follow-up of 30 cases. *Anaesthetist* 1987;**36**:391.
13 Waldman SD, Leak WD, Kennedy LD, *et al.* Intraspinal opioid therapy. In: Patt RB, ed, *Cancer pain.* Philadelphia: JB Lippincott, 1993:285–328.
14 Waldman SD, Feldstein GS, Allen ML. A troubleshooting guide to the subcutaneous epidural implantable reservoir. *J Pain Symptom Management* 1986;**1**:217–22.
15 Meyerson BA. Electrical stimulation of the spinal cord and brain. In: Bonica JJ, ed, *The management of pain,* 2nd edn. Philadelphia: Lea and Febiger, 1990.
16 North R, Ewend M, Lawton M, Kidd D, Piantadosi S. Failed back surgery syndrome: five year follow-up after spinal cord stimulator implantation. *Neurosurgery* 1991;**28**:692–9.
17 Siegfried J, Lazorthes Y. Long term followup of dorsal cord stimulation for chronic pain syndromes aftr multiple lumbar operations. *Appl Neurophysiol* 1982;**45**:201–4.
18 Long DM, Erickson D, Campbell J, North R. Electrical stimulation of the spinal cord and peripheral nerves for pain control. *Appl Neurophysiol* 1981;**44**:207–17.
19 Racz GB, McCarron R, Talboys P. Percutaneous dorsal column stimulator for chronic pain

control. *Spine* 1989;**14**:1–4.

20 North RB. Spinal cord stimulation for intractable pain: indications and technique. *Curr Ther Neurol Surg* 1989;**2**:297–301.

21 Jacobs M, Jorning P, Beckers R, *et al*. Foot salvage and improvement of microvascular flow as the result of epidural spinal cord electrical stimulation. *J Vasc Surg* 1990;**12**:354–60.

22 Waisbrod H, Panhans CH. Direct nerve stimulation for painful peripheral neuropathies. *J Bone Joint Surg* 1985;**67B**:470–2.

23 Cosman ER, Nashold BD, Ovelmann-Levitt J. Theoretical aspects of radiofrequency lesions in the dorsal root entry zone. *Neurosurgery* 1984;**15**:945–50.

24 Kline MT. *Stereotactic radiofrequency lesions as part of the management of pain*. Orlando, FL: Paul M Deutsch, 1992.

25 Sluyter ME, Racz GB, eds *Techniques of neurolysis*. Boston: Kluwer Academic, 1989.

26 Sweet WH. The treatment of trigeminal neuralgia (tic douloureux). *New Engl J Med* 1986;**315**:174–7.

27 Cooper IS. *J Neurol Sci* 1965;**2**:493.

28 Amoils SP. The Joule-Thompson Cryoprobe. *Arch Ophthalmol* 1967;**78**:201–7.

29 Lloyd JW, Barnard JDW, Glynn CJ. Cryoanalgesia, a new approach to pain relief. *Lancet* 1976;**2**:932–4.

30 Nelson K, Vincent R, Bourke R. Interoperative intercostal nerve freezing to prevent postthoracotomy pain. *Ann Thorac Surg* 1974;**18**:280–5.

31 Brain D. Non-neoplastic conditions of the throat and nose. In: Holden HB, ed, *Practical cryosurgery*. St Louis: Mosby, 1975.

32 Evans PJD, Lloyd JW, Green CJ. Cryoanalgesia: the response to alterations in freeze cycle and temperature. *Br J Anaesth* 1981;**53**:1121–7.

33 Sunderland S. *Nerves and nerve injuries*, 2nd edn. London: Churchill Livingstone, 1978.

34 Kalichman MW, Myers RR. Behavioral and electrophysiological recovery following cryogenic nerve injury. *Exp Neurol* 1987;**96**:692–702.

35 Bald WB. A helium gas probe for use in cryosurgery. *Cryobio* 1984;**21**:570–3.

36 Barnard JDW, Lloyd JW, Glynn CJ. Cryosurgery in the management of intractable facial pain. *Br J Oral Surg* 1978–79;**16**:135–41.

37 Goss AN. Cryoneurotomy for intractable temporomandibular joint pain. *Br J Oral Maxillofac Surg* 1988;**26**:26–31.

38 Duthie AM. Pituitary cryoablation. *Anaesthesia* 1983;**38**:495–7.

39 Schuster GD. The use of cryoanalgesia in the painful facet syndrome. *Neurol Orthop Surg* 1982;**3**:271–4.

40 Kluroya RC, Davenport HT, Jones JG. Cryoanalgesia for pain after herniorrhaphy. *Anaesthesia* 1986;**41**:73–6.

41 Wang JK. Cryoanalgesia for painful peripheral nerve lesions. *Pain* 1985;**22**:191–4.

Index